LINCOLN CHRISTIAN COLLEGE AND SEMINARY

P9-DIH-085

TREATING BIPOLAR DISORDER

Treating
Bipolar Disorder

A CLINICIAN'S GUIDE TO INTERPERSONAL AND SOCIAL RHYTHM THERAPY

Ellen Frank

Series Editor's Note by Jacqueline B. Persons

THE GUILFORD PRESS
New York   London

© 2005 The Guilford Press
A Division of Guilford Publications, Inc.
72 Spring Street, New York, NY 10012
www.guilford.com

All rights reserved

Except as indicated, no part of this book may be reproduced, translated, stored in a retrieval system, or transmitted, in any form or by any means, electronic, mechanical, photocopying, microfilming, recording, or otherwise, without written permission from the Publisher.

Printed in the United States of America

This book is printed on acid-free paper.

Last digit is print number: 9   8   7   6   5   4   3   2   1

LIMITED PHOTOCOPY LICENSE

These materials are intended for use only by qualified mental health professionals.

The Publisher grants to individual purchasers of this book nonassignable permission to reproduce the appendices. This license is limited to you, the individual purchaser, for use with your own clients or students. It does not extend to additional clinicians or practice settings, nor does purchase by an institution constitute a site license. This license does not grant the right to reproduce these materials for resale, redistribution, or any other purposes (including but not limited to books, pamphlets, articles, video- or audiotapes, and handouts or slides for lectures or workshops). Permission to reproduce these materials for these and any other purposes must be obtained in writing from the Permissions Department of Guilford Publications.

Library of Congress Cataloging-in-Publication Data

Frank, Ellen.
   Treating bipolar disorder : a clinician's guide to interpersonal and social rhythm therapy / by Ellen Frank.
      p. cm.—(Guides to individualized evidence-based treatment)
   Includes bibliographical references and index.
   ISBN 1-59385-204-5 (hardcover)
   1. Manic–depressive illness—Treatment.   2. Interpersonal and social rhythm therapy.   I. Title.   II. Series.
   RC516.F73 2005
   616.89′ 5—dc22
                                                            2005007029

To my mom

Nancy Newman Frank, MSW

*who taught me most of what I know about helping people
while we did the dishes*

2862/

113229

About the Author

Ellen Frank, PhD, is Professor of Psychiatry and Psychology at the University of Pittsburgh School of Medicine. She received her doctorate in psychology from the University of Pittsburgh in 1979. Dr. Frank's work focuses on the treatment of mood disorders, with particular emphasis on the prevention of recurrence. She is the author of over 350 journal articles, books, and book chapters.

Series Editor's Note

Psychosocial treatment for bipolar disorder is clearly an idea whose time has come. For too long this disorder has been considered the province of medical professionals who provided pharmacotherapy to treat what was seen as a biological disorder. Fortunately, recent years have seen the development of biopsychosocial models and therapies for bipolar disorder. This volume supplies a long-awaited piece of the puzzle: Ellen Frank's exposition of interpersonal and social rhythm therapy (IPSRT).

This book has several outstanding qualities. The formulation of bipolar disorder that underpins IPSRT weaves biological and psychological factors together in an elegant way to obtain an integrated view of the disorder. Thus, IPSRT proposes that episodes of bipolar disorder result from both psychosocial and biological causes—in particular, from external stressful events, especially interpersonal ones, and from disruptions in biological circadian rhythms. Moreover, these two types of causes interact. Thus, for example, a change of jobs, a life event that is stressful for many reasons, can also exert some of its disrupting effects by changing the individual's daily circadian rhythms in response to his or her needing to get up an hour earlier than usual to accommodate a longer commute.

The interventions of IPSRT flow directly and elegantly out of its biopsychosocial conceptualization. Thus, IPSRT works to treat illness episodes and to prevent future ones by helping patients identify and solve interpersonal problems and to maintain regular daily rhythms. Related to the view of the illness as a biopsychosocial disorder, IPSRT is designed to be done in conjunction with pharmacotherapy for most patients.

IPSRT is evidence-based in several ways. The efficacy of the full therapy and of several of its constituent elements is supported by data from randomized controlled trials. In addition, experimental studies linking stressful life events and circadian rhythm disruption to onset of manic and depressive episodes support the conceptualization of the disorder that underpins the therapy.

IPSRT, as presented here, is also evidence-based in that the therapist uses an empirical approach to the treatment of each case. Treatment starts with careful assessment to obtain a diagnosis and develop an IPSRT case formulation that describes the particular interpersonal problems, rhythm disruptions, and mood disorder symptoms that are characteristic of the patient at hand. The formulation guides the therapist's selection of interventions to address the interpersonal problems and rhythm disruptions in order to alleviate the current symptoms and prevent future episodes of illness. As therapy proceeds, the therapist works with the patient to monitor the process and progress of the therapy carefully and make changes as needed, in an empirical and hypothesis-testing way.

Finally, this book displays Ellen Frank's clinical and personal wisdom and her compassion and caring for the patients who struggle with this debilitating disorder. It is truly a privilege to have the opportunity to learn from her that is provided by this book.

JACQUELINE B. PERSONS, PhD
San Francisco Bay Area Center
for Cognitive Therapy

Acknowledgments

Many people contributed to the development of interpersonal and social rhythm therapy (IPSRT) and to the completion of this book. Thanks are due to Thomas Detre, MD, who had a vision of an empirical science of clinical psychiatry and the courage to try to teach that science to an English teacher with absolutely no background in the area, and thus launched me on a career path that led ultimately to the development of IPSRT. Jonathan Himmelhoch, MD, introduced me to the world of clinical care of persons suffering from bipolar disorder and how to understand them. Cindy Ehlers, PhD, had the insights that led to the elaboration of the social *zeitgeber* theory of mood disorders and, with support from the MacArthur Foundation, Joseph Flaherty, MD, and Timothy Monk, PhD, became our primary collaborators in the development of the Social Rhythm Metric, without which it would be hard to imagine IPSRT as it is.

An extraordinary team of research clinicians participated in the Maintenance Therapies in Bipolar Disorder study in which we tested the efficacy of IPSRT, including Gay Herrington, PhD, Kathy Reilly, PhD, Lee Wolfson, MEd, PhD, Lyn Silberman, MSW, Paula Moreci, MSW, Kelly Wells, MSW, and Sue Morris, MSW. I am particularly grateful to Debra Frankel, ACSW, and Steve Carter, PhD, who piloted and developed IPSRT along with me and who contributed many of the case examples in this book. Holly Swartz, MD, came later to the enterprise, but has also had a major role in shaping the final product. Throughout the process, the encouragement and support of David Miklowitz, PhD, who was working in parallel on the development of a family intervention for patients with bipolar disorder, has been a sustaining force.

Special thanks are due to my editors, Kitty Moore of The Guilford Press and Jacqueline B. Persons, PhD, for their extraordinarily wise and kind critiques of each earlier draft and to Patricia Darin for the care with which she prepared the final manuscript.

Most of all, I am grateful to my husband, colleague, and collaborator, David J. Kupfer, MD, for his brilliant insights about the interplay of biological and social factors in understanding the course of bipolar disorder and, therefore, how we might best treat this complex illness, and for his unflagging faith in me and my ability to develop IPSRT and show that it works.

Contents

Introduction

Where IPSRT Came From

Interpersonal and social rhythm therapy (IPSRT) was conceived in a single day; actually, in a single flash of recognition on July 14, 1990. For the previous 10 years I had been working on a long-term maintenance treatment study testing the prophylactic value of interpersonal psychotherapy for individuals with recurrent unipolar depression. In preparation for the study, I, a committed cognitive therapist, had learned Klerman, Weissman, Rounsaville, and Chevron's (1984) interpersonal psychotherapy (IPT) and had been amazed by the power of this deceptively simple approach to the treatment of depression. There's no zealot like a convert. By 1989 I had become a convert to IPT.

As part of our study, our research group was conducting family psychoeducational workshops in an effort to recruit the family members of our study participants as adjunct members of the treatment team. We believed that if family members truly understood that depression was a real and potentially fatal medical illness, if they could see more clearly how patients suffered, if they understood the purpose of the study we were conducting and how what we learned might eventually benefit their family member, then they could be partners in the treatment and research enterprise. This was a fairly radical idea in psychiatry at the time, but it was just that radical idea that appealed to the members of the National Depressive and Manic–Depressive Association (NDMDA; now the Depression and Bipolar Support Alliance).

On that fateful July 14th, which happened to be my 46th birthday, the NDMDA had invited me to speak at its national convention about family involvement in treatment. Because of the flight schedule, I had to fly into Chicago early in the morning even though my talk wasn't scheduled until after lunch. Like most other clinicians who did little direct work with patients who had bipolar disorder, I had thought that bipolar disorder was a problem solved. It took only 5 hours at the NDMDA convention to see how wrong I was!

I began my day by going to see a performance of a group called the New York Mental Health Players. Their performance consisted of a series of vignettes illustrating problems in the life of patients with bipolar disorder. Following each of these vignettes, there was an opportunity for audience comment and discussion. What became apparent during that discussion was the extraordinarily high level of stigma associated with bipolar disorder and how much the NDMDA members in the audience had suffered from it. I remember one woman who had been a nurse who reported being fired by her head nurse when she mentioned that she was taking lithium.

Also impressive was the tremendous disparity between the educational attainment of most of the people there that morning and their current employment status. The audience seemed to be filled with PhDs who were now barely getting by as cab drivers, accountants who were working as clerks in discount drug stores, and other highly trained professionals who didn't even have jobs.

I sat down to lunch with several members of the NDMDA in a beautiful setting on the lawn of the Northwestern University campus, but the conversation I heard was in stark contrast to the brightness of that beautiful July day. Members complained of being discouraged by their psychiatrists from participating in activities that were important to them, such as marathon running, rather than being helped to try to manage the complexities of such endeavors while taking lithium. They talked about the poor quality of their treatment and their clinicians' failure to understand that they needed more than just drugs.

As I was about to give my talk, I stopped in the ladies' room, where I overheard a conversation among three member/volunteers who were discussing how effectively the emergency hospitalization protocol for the conference had been working. Although the conference was only in its second day, three conferees, probably overstimulated by the intensity of the experience, had already needed to be hospitalized.

I arrived at the room where my presentation was scheduled to be held with the normal presenter's fantasy (the room will be empty), only to find that not only was every seat in the room taken, but that individuals with bipolar disorder and their family members were lining the back of the auditorium, sitting in the aisles, and even at the base of the stage. Clearly, family involvement in treatment was something these folks wanted to hear about.

During the next hour and a half, I got a crash course in how desperate these patients and their family members were for attention to the psychosocial issues associated with bipolar disorder, how much they longed for accurate information about the disorder, and how critically important family member involvement was to the successful treatment of manic–depressive illness. By the time I left that auditorium, literally every person in the room was on his or her feet. The intensity of feeling surrounding their needs was palpable. I knew that if I didn't exit the auditorium quickly, I would never make my plane home. So, feeling a little like a rock star being pursued by fans to the door of my limousine (absent the paparazzi), I did my very best to answer as many questions as I could while scurrying through the hallways to the car that was waiting for me.

As the door to the limousine closed and I looked back at the dozen or so people who had accompanied me all the way to my car, I knew with absolute certainty that I needed to dedicate the next decade of my life to doing better by these patients and their family members. No sooner were the words formed in my head than I knew exactly what to do: Combine IPT with a social rhythm regulation treatment.

For several years prior, colleagues at the Western Psychiatric Institute and Clinic and in the MacArthur Foundation Research Network on the Psychobiology of Depression and I had been theorizing about the relationship between *social zeitgebers* (that is, timegivers or timekeepers—think of a metronome) and unipolar disorder. In that moment in the limo I suddenly realized that our theory applied more to bipolar disorder than to unipolar. I also realized that designing a behavioral treatment component to help patients establish and maintain regular social rhythms would not be hard at all, although persuading patients and family members to do it might be a bit of a challenge.

I came home that evening to a huge welcome-the-new-residents party that was taking place in our own backyard. I had only a few seconds to tell my husband and colleague, David Kupfer, about this new idea before needing to play hostess to 18 anxious new residents and their spouses and children. But that night before we went to bed, we sketched out IPSRT on the back of an envelope. All the rest has been elaboration and experience.

The treatment we developed built on the essential components of IPT: taking a history of the patient's illness, educating the patient about the disorder, managing the mood symptoms, learning about the interpersonal realm of the patient's life and its relationship to his or her mood disorder, and intervening to ameliorate existing interpersonal problems and prevent new ones. The major difference between IPSRT and most other modifications of Klerman and colleagues' (1984) original interpersonal psychotherapy is the addition of a large behavior modification component focused on the social rhythms or routines of the patient's life.

My colleagues and I had argued in papers we had published in the late 1980s (Ehlers, Frank, & Kupfer, 1988; Ehlers, Kupfer, Frank, & Monk, 1993) that the major mood disorders (major depression and bipolar disorder) reflected, among other things, a disruption in circadian rhythms, a disturbance in the body's clock. Think about how many of the symptoms of these two disorders are functions that have a regular 24-hour rhythm: sleep (and waking), hunger, energy, ability to concentrate, even mood itself. Furthermore, we said that external social factors, like the time we need to be at work, the time the family normally has dinner, the time a favorite TV show ends, help to set the body's clock. When social factors function in this way, they become social *zeitgebers*. We had also argued that changes or interferences in social routines, which we termed *zeitstörers* (or time disturbers), could disrupt the body's clock and destroy the body's naturally synchronized rhythms. We concluded that, in those who were vulnerable to mood disorders, it was the loss of social *zeitgebers* (timekeepers) or the appearance of *zeitstörers* (disrupters) that led to new illness episodes (depression or mania).

During that flash in the limo, I knew it would be relatively easy to borrow some of the scheduling and monitoring techniques of cognitive therapy and refashion them for the purpose of helping patients to establish and maintain regular social rhythms. I also realized that such efforts would fit very naturally with at least three of the four interpersonal problem areas that form the foundation of the interpersonal work in IPT for unipolar depression: resolving an unresolved grief experience, negotiating a transition in a major life role, and resolving a role dispute with a significant other. Thus, IPSRT became a treatment that seeks to improve on the outcomes that are usually obtained with pharmacotherapy alone for patients suffering from bipolar I disorder by integrating efforts to regularize their social rhythms (in the hope of protecting their circadian systems from disruption) with efforts to improve the quality of their interpersonal relationships and social role functioning. The addition of a new problem area, grief for the lost healthy self, to the four original IPT problem areas is aimed at increasing acceptance of the illness and improving treatment adherence in a patient group for which these are both difficult issues.

When we set out to develop a psychotherapeutic intervention that could enhance or complement drug therapy for manic–depressive illness, one of the questions we asked ourselves was, "What kinds of things do first-rate clinicians do with patients who have this disorder in addition to prescribing appropriate medications?" We realized that most expert pharmacotherapists in the area of bipolar disorder always recommended a series of lifestyle changes in addition to careful adherence to the medication regimen they prescribed. Furthermore, we realized that these lifestyle modifications were all consistent with a model of the illness that posits physiological instability as central to the pathology of bipolar I disorder. Thus, our rationale for IPSRT had a foundation in a more general understanding of the pathophysiology of all recurrent mood disorders and in the research literature on recurrent unipolar and bipolar disorder.

In the time since my trip to that NDMDA national convention, with the help of dozens of colleagues and hundreds of patients, IPSRT has evolved from a fledgling idea to a fully elaborated treatment. Yet, as we continue to learn from our patients, IPSRT continues to evolve. As you read this book and use this treatment, you will undoubtedly think of additional ways to help your patients develop and maintain supportive interpersonal relationships and satisfying social roles while leading lives that are characterized by sufficient regularity and routine to reduce the risk of new episodes of illness.

ONE

The Patients

At 18, Jill's future could not have seemed brighter. She had just been accepted into the prestigious college she and her parents had always thought would be perfect for her. She had a large circle of bright and trusted friends, a wonderful boyfriend who would be attending a college nearby, and parents who adored and supported her. True, she had had a few tough semesters in high school, times when her boundless energy and enthusiasm seemed to fail her, when getting out of bed in the morning was just incredibly difficult, when simply deciding whether to wear the white turtleneck or the gray one seemed to take hours, when her usually rapt attention would drift and finishing a paragraph in her history text or a brief poem for English would require that she read and reread and reread again, when nothing seemed like much fun to this usually exuberant young woman. These periods puzzled her parents, but they simply attributed it to adolescent moodiness, especially in light of the fact that when spring came she always seemed to manage to pull herself (and her grades) up by her own bootstraps.

Jill experienced some difficulty in adapting to the natural disorder of college life, especially as compared with the orderly home life she had known: dinners between 6:30 and 7:00, lights out throughout the house by midnight, everyone up and at the breakfast table by 6:45, regular runs with her dad each Saturday at 10:00, and church every Sunday, followed by a big family gathering at her grandmother's. Sensing that she felt better when things were more like they had been at home, after her first year at college, Jill found a roommate who shared her desire for order in the midst of the chaos, who didn't think that pulling all-nighters was cool, and who was willing to hang a Do Not Disturb sign on their door when they wanted to get some sleep.

Graduating as a Phi Beta Kappa, Jill had her choice of graduate programs. She chose one in which she thought she could shine while still having some time to pursue a personal life. Continuing her apparently charmed existence, she left grad school with both a PhD and a Mrs. She and her new husband, also an English professor-in-the-making, were fortunate to find positions in the same Eastern city, and their life seemed set—until the birth of their first child 2 years later. Within 5 days of delivering, Jill turned into someone neither of them knew: sobbing hysterically one moment, grandiose the next, she often made no sense. She was convinced that her little boy had the "mark of Satan" and had no qualms about telling her pediatrician, who had declared the child perfectly fine, that her baby was doomed. Fortunately, the pediatrician recognized her excited, psychotic mixed state as a postpartum psychosis and referred her for psychiatric treatment. Over the objections of her husband, her parents and, of course, Jill herself, the psychopharmacologist to whom she had been referred insisted that Jill be hospitalized involuntarily. Within a few days, with the aid of massive amounts of lithium and a whiff of a typical neuroleptic, Jill appeared much like her old self.

Her psychiatrist tried to explain what the events of the last week meant in terms of long-term prognosis, but "manic–depressive illness" and "bipolar disorder" were not words that Jill or anyone in her family wanted to hear. "No one in our family has ever had anything like this. Manic–depressive illness is a genetic disorder. We get heart disease, but not anything like this." Nonetheless, her psychiatrist insisted that, given her history of mild seasonal mood swings since adolescence, her history of generally good adjustment and social relations prior to this episode, the appearance of a first episode of psychosis immediately postpartum, and, most important, the fact that she responded quickly and completely to treatment with lithium and a very small dose of antipsychotic medication, all the indicators pointed in the direction of a diagnosis of bipolar disorder.

As the months passed, Jill resumed her teaching, again to high praise. She was caring for her child with great affection and little effort and still found time for a full and rich life with her husband. The whole bizarre episode that followed her son's birth became a kind of aberration in an otherwise perfect existence, something she and her family just wanted to forget. She kept finding reasons to cancel her appointments with her psychopharmacologist. She had so many more important, more meaningful things to do. Eventually she ran out of lithium . . . and, contrary to her doctor's dire predictions, nothing seemed to happen.

All went well for the next few years; her child, her career, and her marriage flourished. When Jill's little boy was 3, her sister-in-law, to whom Jill was very close, became pregnant. Having taken the winter quarter off to write that year, Jill volunteered to go to Seattle to help her care for the new baby. Within days of her arrival she realized what a mistake she had made. There really wasn't space for her and her son in her brother and sister-in-law's cramped apartment. Neither of them had ever been big on regular routines, and with the new baby, nothing ever happened on schedule. Jill found it nearly impossible to calm her son, to feed him on anything like a regular basis, or to get any reading done at night when the entire household seemed to be in perpetual motion. And it never stopped raining! So she and that ball of energy that was her son could never escape. Soon she found herself feeling like she had during those awful times in high school. Worst of all, she could never really talk to her husband. Between the 3-hour time difference and the lack of privacy, she felt totally isolated from her "rock," as she often called him. By the time Jill got back home, she was in a nearly immobilizing depression. Writing was impossible. She couldn't even read more than a paragraph without losing her train of thought. She dragged herself through her days, barely managing to get something like dinner on the table by the time her husband returned from teaching. In fact, many nights he came home to find her just sitting on the sofa, staring at the TV, surprised that he was home already. Neither Jill nor her husband knew how to explain what was happening, and neither saw any relationship between this immobility and the experience Jill had had right after their son was born.

After much self-torture and recrimination, Jill came to realize that she could not possibly return to the university when the spring quarter began and asked for a temporary leave of absence. She would never go back.

It took almost a year, but finally, Jill's depression lifted. She, her husband, and her family made a million excuses for what had happened: She had pushed herself too hard too soon, she wasn't really cut out for the competitive nastiness of academic life, she was too sensitive a soul, she was too devoted to her students and her family and had too much difficulty putting her own career ahead of their needs and the conflict finally got to her, and so on.

Maybe she would do better in a kinder, less demanding atmosphere and still be able to experience the joy of teaching literature. Without much difficulty, she found a position at a small private girl's high school. The school was thrilled to have someone of her caliber teaching their juniors and seniors, the other teachers were warm and friendly, and the students were any teacher's dream: bright, inquisitive, and always prepared. She made next to nothing, but she was happy: "This will be just fine until my kids are grown. Then I'll go back to the university grind."

With her life more or less back in order, Jill and her husband decided to have another child. The pregnancy went well, she felt fine, and she taught until the week before she delivered their second son, just as her summer vacation was starting. Within a day of her return from the hospital, however, Jill's husband began to see ominous signs of a repeat of their prior postbirth experience. He tried to contact Jill's former psychopharmacologist, but she had moved. He didn't know where to turn. He was afraid to say anything to Jill's parents and just hoped he was being unduly skittish. By the time of her first postpartum visit to the pediatrician, however, there was no denying that she was even more ill than she had been after her first son's birth. And he felt he could count on their pediatrician to confront Jill about it.

This time with the support of her parents, Jill's husband was able to persuade her to go into the hospital voluntarily . . . though just barely. Once she was there, she nearly signed herself out on three occasions before the medications began to take effect. Again, Jill responded well to the combination of lithium and a typical neuroleptic and was home within 10 days.

Unable to deny that there was a pattern to her illness, Jill committed herself to her treatment, going regularly to see her new psychopharmacologist and taking her medicine like clockwork. In the fall she returned to her beloved teaching job and seemed to manage very well for the next several years. Her boys were thriving, but she and her husband really wanted a daughter as well. They consulted her doctor, who felt that with a very slow taper of her lithium—that was all she had taken since her last baby was about 6 weeks old—and reinstitution of her medication a few weeks before delivery, they had a good chance of averting a third postpartum episode.

What he hadn't counted on was that Jill would miscarry in her 5th month. The rapid hormonal shift and the emotional impact of the miscarriage were more than enough to send her into another episode of psychosis and back into the hospital, but this time she did not show her typical quick response to medication. Her doctor tried one thing after another, but nothing seemed to bring her delusions or manic excitement under control. Her husband, who had never before been the focus of her psychotic thinking, was devastated when she accused him of having an affair with one of his colleagues while she was "locked up in this snake pit." He was struggling to manage his teaching and other departmental responsibilities, and their two rambunctious little boys, and get to the hospital to see her every night, so her vicious accusations, loud enough for the whole inpatient unit to hear, put him over the edge. He would go home each night and replay the horror scenes in the hospital in his head and then replay them all day when he should have been writing, or reading students' essays, or playing with his boys.

Finally, Jill's treatment team decided that only electroconvulsive therapy (ECT) held any real promise for bringing her mania under control. Her husband was desperate for anything that would stop the maltreatment from Jill that he experienced each night. Still, there was enough of a thread of a relationship left between them that he was able to convince her that this might be a way out of the hospital. After the first ECT treatment, he could see a difference. This was going to work. They would return to their happy enough life. The daughter they had dreamed of was unimportant as compared with just getting back to some semblance of normality. And he was right: The ECT did bring Jill's mania completely under control, but she came home a fragile, tentative woman whom he hardly knew. By turns silent and irritable, she was difficult to engage in conversation, let alone in any physical intimacy. They began to fight . . . over everything: the boys, when to have supper, how much time he spent at his office (maybe she still thought he was having an affair), how messy the house was, everything.

As the fall approached, Jill, who had had to take a year's leave from her teaching job, made an appointment to see her department head and make plans for the upcoming term. Only then did he tell Jill that her position had been filled by an excellent substitute whom the school was reluctant to let go. They were terribly sorry. They knew the miscarriage must have been very hard for her. She drove home, not even knowing how she had arrived there, feeling as if her last anchor had been pulled and she was totally adrift. She thought briefly about going to "talk" to someone but, hearing her mother's voice echoing in her head, knew that "we just don't do that in our family. We handle our problems ourselves."

Jill realized that she was much too fragile to manage the stress of teaching in the big public high school where she might have been able to get a position. Instead, she took a job in a children's bookstore near her home. At least they were willing to give her hours that would allow her to get home before her boys, get dinner ready, begin to take care of the house like she used to. But none of it seemed to matter. Her husband remained distant, they fought all the time, her boys were out of control, the household was in chaos. One night her husband just didn't come home. In some ways, it was a relief.

The next day he came to the bookstore and asked if she could take a coffee break. At the coffee shop, he told her he had been out walking the campus all night, trying to figure out a way to tell her that he just needed a peaceful place to go home to. She and the boys would never have to worry, he would always take care of them, but he needed to move out. The "rock" needed some time to regroup.

*   *   *   *

At the point that Jill appeared for treatment with IPSRT, she and her husband had been separated for more than 3 years and their divorce was imminent. She had not worked since the day her husband came to the bookstore. She kept telling herself she'd go back, but she never did. Finally, the bookstore closed and she couldn't think of any place that would want her. She was barely getting by financially, but knew her soon-to-be ex could not afford more on his university salary. Her parents couldn't (or wouldn't) help. They really didn't understand why she wasn't still at her own university job. Her children were beginning to have problems in school, and she was at a loss to know what to do about it. Summers were worse. All three of them would wander aimlessly through the days, never going to bed at a reasonable time, getting up whenever they felt like it. Finally, she decided that she just wasn't going to go through another school year with them like the last one. She needed some help getting her life together. She couldn't remember the last time she had spent any time, or wanted to spend any time, with a friend. She wasn't exactly depressed, but she had never really snapped back after her last hospitalization. It seemed as though the doctor could never get her meds quite right . . . and every time she started to feel something like her old energy and enthusiasm come back, they would both panic and agree that she needed more. What had happened to that brilliant future that seemed so assured just a dozen or so summers ago?

Jill's history is typical of those who suffer from manic–depressive illness in many respects and, unfortunately, especially typical of those patients who never receive any sort of psychosocial treatment or psychoeducation. Her early life was characterized by great energy, intellectual promise, and good social relationships. The quality of her early upbringing, including a warm and supportive family that led an orderly existence, kept her protected from most manifestations of mood disorder, with the exception of some relatively mild and brief episodes of seasonal depression that went essentially unrecognized. Her own maturity, good sense, and wisdom about what she needed to function well (a regular routine, sufficient sleep, structure, etc.) protected her during college, graduate school, and the early years of her marital and professional life. In Jill's case, it took the massive hormonal and circadian challenge of parturition to bring about the expression of her bipolar illness. Once she became ill, some of the very things that had protected her earlier—the absence of any apparent mood disorder in her immediate family, the basic rigidity of her parents, her naiveté as well as that of her parents and husband about psychiatric illness—eventually proved to be her downfall. Had she (and they) received more in the way of psychoeducation about mood disorder, both her subsequent manias and her severe depression might have been averted. She had had the good fortune of responding well to an initial treatment regimen that was relatively uncomplicated and kept her symptoms under good control. However, at the beginning neither she nor her family had really understood or accepted the lifelong nature of her illness and its propensity to recur. Had she received psychotherapy focused on the management of her illness and her interpersonal life in the context of that illness, she might not have made the trip to Seattle or been so puzzled by what was happening to her marriage. But, here, even her psychopharmacologist failed to see what was needed. In the absence of any kind of psychosocial intervention, many of those who suffer from bipolar disorder find themselves on the deteriorative course that characterized Jill's life, a course from which it can be very difficult to recover.

Still, Jill brought many strengths to her IPSRT treatment. Perhaps most important, she was highly motivated to change the direction of her life. In addition, she was intelligent, verbal, and reasonably insightful. Although not the person she had been a decade earlier, she retained many of the social skills she had had as a young woman. Finally, because her illness did not begin until she was an adult, she had an idea of what it meant to be fully functional even though it had been many years since she was able to do so.

Jill's IPSRT therapist began by taking a history of her bipolar illness, going all the way back to her seasonal mood changes in high school. Together they created a timeline in which her episodes, her treatments, and any life circumstances that seemed to be associated with the onset of symptoms were represented, along with her work and marital status. Her therapist pointed out how important challenges to her circadian system and changes in her hormonal state seemed to be connected to the onsets of her episodes. He also pointed out how much better she seemed to function when she was in a regular routine. He queried her about the various medications she had taken over the course of her illness, trying to understand what had worked best for her. He then completed what we call the "interpersonal inventory," an informal review of all the relationships that were currently important to Jill and all the relationships that had been important to her in the past. He discovered how socially isolated this once well-integrated woman had become. In taking the illness history and the interpersonal inventory he was also able to see the clear decline in her work functioning. At their fourth session, he discussed the IPSRT problem areas with Jill and together they agreed that first she needed to grieve for her lost healthy self and former life as a functioning professional and wife. They talked about the fact that she really had not fully made the transition to being single or to being a single parent and decided that this would be a later focus of their work. First, though, they needed to concentrate on getting Jill and her boys into some sort of regular routine. Fortunately, Jill's therapist didn't need to do much to convince her that she would feel better if she were on a regular schedule. That was something she knew already. He gave her the Social Rhythm Metric to complete before their next session. When she returned the following week, he could see that the time at which she was getting up in the mornings varied by as much as 3 hours a day. Knowing that a person's "good morning time" tends to set the body's clock, he concentrated on having Jill get up at a regular time each day. Because it was summer and the boys didn't need to be at school, he chose 9:00 A.M. as the target, thinking that later in the summer he could help Jill work her way toward an earlier wake-up time. He also suggested that she focus on making a real breakfast for herself and the boys and eating breakfast as a family each morning, thinking that that would be good for Jill's self-esteem, further help to set her clock, and bring a bit of needed stability to the boys' lives. At each visit, he praised her progress and encouraged her to stick with what was a difficult challenge for her. He inquired regularly about her symptoms and about her response to the new medications his colleague had prescribed, including any side effects she might be experiencing. Once she was on a modestly regular schedule, he began to help her grieve for the young professor of such high promise and for all that she had hoped to become. He gently helped her to see how her once supportive parents had subsequently failed her by mostly denying her illness. He asked Jill if she thought it might ever be useful for the four of them to meet together, and when she tentatively said yes, he tucked away the idea of a conjoint psychoeducational session as something he would attempt to schedule in a month or two when Jill was feeling stronger. He took a more careful history of the marriage and what its loss had meant to her. He tried to understand what kind of life Jill wanted now and how much of what she wanted she might be capable of having. Very, very gradually over the ensuing months Jill came to accept her illness as a challenge she might be able to master and her life as a single mother as one that might offer satisfactions. When the therapist did attempt the conjoint educational session with her parents, he realized that they were just too uptight, angry, and disappointed to be able to be a support to Jill without entering into treatment themselves, something he thought it unlikely they would ever do. After that, Jill's therapist helped her to reconnect with other, less judgmental sources of support and to garner some new ones. He kept his expectations for her modest and tried to convey those modest expectations to Jill. By Halloween, Jill was able to host a small neighborhood party for her boys' friends and some of their parents. Her boys were enormously pleased, and Jill was pleased with herself, perhaps for the first time in years. Whether she would ever be able to go back to working was a question they left open, for now focusing just on keeping Jill's mood stable, her routines regular, and her boys' functioning at home and at school on a steady course of improvement.

In some ways, Tad was more fortunate than Jill, even though the beginnings of their stories sound similar. At 18, Tad's future also seemed incredibly bright. A gifted artist from the time he was a little boy, he had been accepted to one of the foremost fine arts colleges in the nation. He was going to have an opportunity to study painting with a man whose work was world renowned, despite the fact that Tad had grown up in a tiny town in Alabama, had never been in a real museum, and had never seen a great painting except in the art books his mother had borrowed from the library where she worked. His interests had made him an outcast as early as junior high, but knowing that he would finally get to do what he had dreamed of doing for as long as he could remember eclipsed all the suffering he had experienced in high school. And there had been quite a lot: months when he was so sad he could hardly speak, moments when, out of the blue, he was consumed with heart-stopping anxiety so terrifying he was certain he was going to die, days when he was so irritable that even his sainted mother lost her seemingly endless patience with him and he felt utterly abandoned in the world.

At college he found not one, not two, but dozens of soul mates, people who seemed to care just as intensely as he did and were willing to talk about their passions from the minute classes ended until the sun came up the next morning. And then there were the museums! Just a subway ride away, there was a veritable feast for the eyes, the intellect. Whenever he wanted, he could take off for an hour and see a real Picasso, or Rembrandt, or van Gogh, and unlike the way he was in high school, he seemed to have boundless energy. Indeed, within a few weeks he found he really didn't need to sleep. He could spend all afternoon in the museums and almost all night talking with his classmates, and when he finally made his way back to his room, he still had energy enough to do his homework and finish his projects—brilliantly! The wildest, most original ideas kept coming to him, day after day, week after week. The sunshine on the minerals in the cement of the sidewalk appeared to him like van Gogh's starry nights. As he walked back to his dorm just before dawn, the shadows of the twisted old trees on the campus had all the weight and intensity of one Michelangelo's dying slaves. He had never experienced anything like it! When it came time to plan his first-semester final project, he was a bit secretive with his advisor, who, because Tad's work to date had been so exceptional, decided to just wait and see what this brilliant young kid came up with. To his advisor's horror, what Tad presented as his project was a complex and visually stunning installation, which he had completed in a single night in the men's gymnasium, made entirely of women's underwear, stolen one piece at a time from the drawers of his dorm mates. The text he wrote to accompany his exhibition was completely incomprehensible, like something written by a madman. Neither his advisor nor the administration nor the women from whom he had taken the underwear were the least amused. When interviewed the following day by the dean, it was immediately apparent that this was not just some drug-induced joke. Tad was a seriously ill young man.

Immediately referred for treatment of his mania by the school administration, Tad presented numerous challenges to his IPSRT treatment team. Naturally, he at first denied that there was anything wrong with him or that he had any need for treatment. Once the team was able to begin treatment in earnest, his mania proved very hard to control pharmacologically, and, although he was chronologically 18, his social development was found to be more like that of a 14-year-old. He was alone in a big city with no real support system other than his treatment team. Sending him back to the dormitory, where overstimulation and easy access to drugs had already proven to be a major problem, was not an option. Together with Tad, his treatment team worked out a housing and scholastic plan that would eventually allow him to reenter school on a part-time and, later, full-time basis. In the interim, he would enter an assisted-living facility where medications were dosed by the staff and take a part-time job as a clerk at a 7-Eleven.

It took two more severe episodes of mania, hours of psychotherapy, and the unwavering support and encouragement of his treatment team, but Tad finally accepted the need for ongoing pharmacotherapy. Unfortunately, the only medications that controlled his symptoms made Tad's hands tremble so that he had to give up his dream of becoming a painter. However, like Matisse, he learned (with his advisor's encouragement and support) to work in other media when he could no longer create in the way that was most natural to him. It took 6 years, but Tad did finish school and, during that time, matured about twice 6 years. Much of his psychotherapy focused on grieving for all the dreams he had once had—of doing great work, of traveling and studying abroad, of making full use of his gifts—and on doing all he could to keep his symptoms under control. This included keeping to a very regular schedule, getting sufficient sleep, avoiding excessive stimulation, and being sure to get adequate sleep in the social context of fine arts studies (where routine is anathema). By the time Tad was ready to graduate, he had come to accept the numerous limitations his illness placed on him. Rather than remain in a city that always threatened to tempt him with overstimulation and easy access to drugs, he opted to return to the town where he had grown up. Back in Alabama, he knew he could count on the support of his mother and sister should he become ill again. Still a gifted artist and irrepressible art enthusiast, he accepted a position as an elementary art teacher in the same school where his mother serves as librarian (and close observer of any changes in his moods). He adores the children he works with, and they adore him and his enthusiasm. His family doctor prescribes his medications, and both he and his doctor remain in occasional touch with the treatment team that put him on the road to a stable and satisfying life.

Tad's story is a good illustration of what can happen when a very needy, but entirely likable, young patient with bipolar disorder has the good fortune to encounter a skilled and dedicated treatment team early in the course of his illness. From the outset, his team members understood that despite his enormous size (6'3" and over 200 pounds), social grace, and intellectual gifts, he was really a scared little boy alone in a huge city with no skills or other supports to combat his illness. They interpreted his initial denial of his illness and nonadherence to treatment as perfectly normal . . . and told him so. They stuck with him through a series of hospitalizations for mania (when he often treated them despicably) and through the difficult, drawn-out depressions and the suicide threats that followed each of these episodes. By telephone and during his mother's occasional visits, they worked closely with his family members to educate them about what was happening to their beloved Tad, what his illness would mean for both his short-term and long-term plans, and why the medications that made his long-dreamed-of career impossible were necessary for his survival. At each step along the way, they helped him to grieve for what he was losing and congratulated him on what he was accomplishing. To this day, despite the fact that he has not seen the members of his treatment team face-to-face for almost a decade, their approval of his life choices and their interest in his accomplishments remain an important source of pride.

Although Jill and Tad entered treatment at very different stages in their battle with bipolar illness, IPSRT proved to be an appropriate intervention for both of them. In Jill's case it helped her climb out of what seemed to be a morass of symptoms, stress, and unmanageable responsibilities to live a life of dignity, albeit not the life she had foreseen for herself at age 22, but one of which she could be justifiably proud and which provided her children with the stability they needed. In Tad's case, IPSRT was able to set him on a life course that was consistent with the perils his disorder presented if he failed to respect the limitations that it set for him. He, too, found a life of dignity and deep satisfactions, although not those he had anticipated when he first became ill.

Interpersonal and social rhythm therapy (IPSRT) was developed with the late adolescent and adult patient with bipolar I disorder in mind. It has been tested in a randomized clinical trial that included only individuals over the age of 18 with a diagnosis of bipolar I disorder who had experienced at least two past episodes of mania and/or depression. The anecdotal evidence gained from our own pilot studies and from our experience in training therapists in the conduct of IPSRT suggests that it is also an appropriate intervention in younger patients, in individuals who are experiencing only their first or second episode of bipolar depression or mania, and in individuals with bipolar II disorder.

In characterizing the patient for whom the treatment is intended, we refer the reader to the descriptions of manic episode, major depressive episode, and bipolar I disorder provided in the fourth edition of the *Diagnostic and Statistical Manual of Mental Disorders* (DSM-IV; American Psychiatric Association, 2000, pp. 350–355) and to the extensive description of the disorder provided in Goodwin and Jamison's classic 1990 volume, *Manic Depressive Illness*. Briefly, the essential feature of bipolar I disorder is the lifetime experience of an episode of mania. Episodes of depression are usually present in the history as well, but are not a requirement for the official DSM-IV diagnosis. In contrast, the diagnosis of bipolar II disorder requires that the individual have a history of both hypomanic and depressive episodes. Formal diagnostic considerations aside, IPSRT is almost certainly appropriate for any patient with clearly defined and impairing episodes of high and low mood (as opposed to fleeting shifts in mood) that are accompanied by the cognitive and neurovegetative changes associated with mania/hypomania and depression. With respect to mania/hypomania, these changes include inflated self-esteem and grandiose thinking (often reaching delusional levels in mania), reduced need for sleep, increased energy, sexual interest and activity, rapid speech and thought, and increased involvement in pleasurable activities without regard for the consequences such activities might have. With respect to depression, such changes include loss of interest in usually pleasurable activities; decreased energy; increased *or* decreased sleep, appetite, and weight; difficulty in thinking, concentrating, remembering, or making decisions; reduced self-esteem; and thoughts of death or suicide.

Although the epidemiological data suggest that bipolar I disorder (which has a lifetime prevalence of about 1% in most industrialized societies in which it has been studied) is equally likely to afflict men and women, our experience and that of our colleagues is that about two thirds of those who seek voluntary treatment for this condition are female. The female-to-male ratio is probably even higher for bipolar II disorder. Both classic manic–depressive illness (bipolar I) and its more attenuated forms (bipolar II, bipolar disorder not otherwise specified [NOS], and cyclothymia) tend to begin in the late teens or early 20s, although patients may suffer for many years or even decades before an appropriate diagnosis is made. Especially if the manias are nonpsychotic, not terribly destructive, or even, in some ways, functional, the bipolar aspect of the illness may be missed unless a very careful history is taken. A group of almost 3,000 individuals participating in a bipolar disorder patient registry that we maintain at the University of Pittsburgh reports that it took, on average, 10 years from their first episode of illness to the time they received a correct diagnosis from a professional (Kupfer, Frank, Grochocinski, Cluss, et al., 2002).

Perhaps more important to the introductory discussion in this chapter is the *nature* of the depressive or manic/hypomanic illness at the time IPSRT is being initiated. As becomes obvious in subsequent chapters, this is an intervention that requires considerable effort and, particularly, effort at change on the patient's part. Thus, IPSRT is intended for individuals whose clinical condition is such that major psychotic symptoms have receded or are absent. Although IPSRT can be started either in the hospital or on an outpatient basis, our experience with this treatment has been almost exclusively with individuals who have already been discharged from the hospital or were not hospitalized in the first place. Because written homework is required, a moderate level of literacy is necessary for participation in IPSRT, at least as it was originally conceptualized. Most of this homework relates to the completion of the Social Rhythm Metric (SRM; Monk, Flaherty, Frank, Hoskinson, & Kupfer, 1990; Monk, Kupfer, Frank, & Ritenour, 1991), a self-monitoring form, originally 17 items in length, for recording the time at which and with whom a series of daily activities are completed. We have recently created a simpler and shorter, five-item version of this self-monitoring device (Monk, Frank, Potts, & Kupfer, 2002) that could almost certainly be adapted to the needs of individuals with very limited literacy. Copies of both versions of the SRM appear in the Appendices (short version, Appendix 1; long version, Appendix 3).

Although both of the case examples at the beginning of this chapter describe individuals of above average intelligence and talent who had high educational attainment, we have engaged individuals of much lower intelligence levels and much lower educational attainment in IPSRT. Even though it is true that the population of individuals who have suffered from bipolar disorder does include some of the world's most gifted persons, there are also many ordinary citizens who must cope with this condition, and IPSRT appears to be able to help them do that.

As noted earlier, IPSRT was developed for use with "adult" patients with manic–depressive illness. The youngest individuals we have treated with IPSRT were 18 years of age at the time they entered treatment. IPSRT, however, could almost certainly be applied to relatively mature late adolescents, especially those whose families can be engaged as "coaches" for the changes the patient is being asked to make. At the upper end of the age spectrum, the oldest patients we have treated with IPSRT to date are those in their 60s. However, we are beginning to try to understand how IPSRT functions in the relatively small population of individuals with classical manic–depressive illness who continue to suffer into their 70s, 80s, and beyond.

Interpersonal and social rhythm therapy was developed with primarily Anglo and African American patients in mind. We have used it with good success with small numbers of patients of Asian, East Indian and Middle Eastern backgrounds, but have essentially no experience in using it with individuals of Hispanic origin. It is clear, however, that interpersonal therapy and the interpersonal aspects of IPSRT are, by their very nature, adaptable to virtually any cultural or subcultural background. In IPT and IPSRT the interpersonal problem areas to be addressed are always conceptualized within the context of the subject's own values with respect to interpersonal roles and relationships. Likewise, the social routines aspect of the treatment makes no particular judgment as to when specific daily routines should occur, but simply emphasizes the importance of regularity of routines in the lives of those who suffer from manic–depressive illness. If breakfast is not taken until after morning prayers are said, or the large meal is eaten at midday, or there is a period of sleep following the midday meal as essential parts of a cultural routine, the treatment is easily able to accommodate these cultural preferences. Thus, in theory at least, IPSRT should be adaptable to a multiplicity of ethnic groups and subcultures.

The chapters that follow describe something about the theories of etiology of bipolar disorder and bipolar episodes and the other treatments that have been shown to be effective in this condition that follow from these theories. We describe our own theoretical stance in detail because it provides the basic rationale for IPSRT. Then we take you through the various elements of assessment and treatment that constitute IPSRT. We also describe other useful interventions that work well as adjuncts to IPSRT and offer some thoughts about the therapeutic relationship in IPSRT and what to do when the treatment does not seem to be helpful. Finally, we discuss the issue of termination or transition to more limited contact with the patient.

An essential foundation for IPSRT is familiarity with Klerman and colleagues' interpersonal psychotherapy (IPT) for unipolar disorder (Klerman et al., 1984; Weissman, Markowitz, & Klerman, 2000). If you are contemplating using IPSRT yourself, you would do well to read one of these two books describing IPT. Although it is very helpful to obtain supervision from an experienced IPT or IPSRT clinician, in many places it may be difficult to find such a person. In the absence of the availability of such supervision, we recommend finding a colleague who shares your interest in practical, present-focused treatments and asking him or her to read through this book, begin to apply IPSRT in his or her practice, and then, using audiotapes of treatment sessions, engage in informal peer supervision with you.

TWO

Empirically Supported Theories of Bipolar Disorder and the Etiology of Bipolar Episodes

Bipolar disorder is a biologically based disorder with multiple psychological components, as well as factors that are reactive to environmental changes. Among psychiatric disorders, bipolar disorder has been long considered one in which physiologic and presumed genetic factors (in the form of a positive family history) play a strong role. Nonetheless, it appears that the timing of individual episodes may be strongly related to environmental and other psychological and psychosocial factors, suggesting an important role for psychosocial treatments in the amelioration of the course of this potentially devastating and sometimes lethal illness.

GENETIC FACTORS

The risk for bipolar I disorder in the relatives of those diagnosed with this condition probably ranges from as high as 60–70% for a monozygotic twin to approximately 2–5% for a grandchild or cousin (Bertelsen, Harvald, & Hauge, 1977; Gershon et al., 1982). Considering that the risk in the general population is between 1 and 2%, this argues strongly for a genetic basis to the disorder. The search for mechanisms of inheritance of manic–depressive illness has led scientists to conclude that it is "a complex genetic disorder," probably consisting of several distinct genetic vulnerability traits. The expression of these traits will ultimately be transmitted across generations and sets up a level of risk for developing the full syndrome at some point in the life cycle. It is thought, however, that early-onset bipolar disorder is associated with a greater genetic penetrance. That is, those with the most genetic vulnerability factors or the densest loading of ill relatives are likely to display the syndrome at an especially early age. The biological manifestation of these genetic factors may be found in neurotransmitter abnormalities or circadian dysregulation, two examples of how the biological expression affects the timing and onset of the disorder and of episodes of illness.

NEUROTRANSMISSION THEORIES

Bipolar disorder or manic–depressive illness was probably the first psychiatric condition to be associated with the term "chemical imbalance." The idea that something was seriously awry in the brain chemistry of those who suffered from bipolar disorder has held sway for nearly a century and has been the subject of serious scientific investigation since the discovery that chemical agents could have dramatic effects on the symptomatology of the illness.

The array of disparate medications indicated for bipolar disorder, and the utility of these pharmacological agents in the treatment of either manic or depressive episodes, hint at the complexities underlying the biochemical basis for the disorder. For manic episodes, lithium carbonate, valproic acid (an anticonvulsant), and antipsychotic agents are all suggested as first-line treatments; lithium and lamotrigine (another anticonvulsant) are suggested as first-line treatments for bipolar depression, after which antidepressants such as the selective serotonin reuptake inhibitors (SSRIs) bupropion and venlafaxine are employed (American Psychiatric Association, 2002) in combination with lithium or another so-called mood stabilizer. For mood stabilization between acute episodes, lithium, anticonvulsants, and antispsychotics are all used frequently.

Probing the pharmacological effects of these disparate agents, research has focused on the common underlying mechanisms that hypothetically may account for the efficacy of these diverse treatments. Early research examined the monaminergic system (see Halbreich & Montgomery, 2000). Subsequently, other neurotransmitters such as gamma-aminobutyric acid (GABA) and acetylcholine, and signal transduction networks such as the cyclic adenosine monophate/protein kinase A, the phosphoinositide/protein kinase C, G protein, and calcium signaling networks have been explored (Manji & Lenox, 1999). Undoubtedly, the complex interplay among these diverse systems accounts for the complex clinical presentation of bipolar disorder and the differing responses to pharmacological agents.

The trait abnormality of low serotonin function in both the depressive and manic phases points to a dysregulation in this system as well (Goodwin & Jamison, 1990). The ramifications of altered serotonergic function are complicated by the various serotonin receptor subtypes, their distribution in the central nervous system, and their modulation of other neurotransmitter systems such as the catecholamines (dopamine and norepinephrine) (Goodwin & Jamison, 1990; Manji & Lenox, 1999). A plausible role for catecholamines in depression, hypomania, and mania has also been hypothesized (Goodwin & Jamison, 1990). Increased norepinephrine correlates with hypomanic symptoms such as euphoria and grandiosity, and increased dopamine correlates with manic and psychotic symptoms (Goodwin & Jamison, 1990).

In the raphe nucleus and substantia nigra, noradrenergic neurons inhibit dopamine release, and therefore it has been proposed that depression itself, with decreased norepinephrine, predisposes individuals to excessive dopamine release and a switch into mania (Goodwin & Jamison, 1990). The idea that dopamine is implicated in the onset of bipolar mania gains credence through the ability of the dopamine precursor L-dopa, amphetamines, and dopamine agonists to produce hypomanic and manic symptoms in bipolar subjects (Yatham et al., 2002). In addition, D_2 receptor antagonists are efficacious in the treatment of mania.

The role of GABA has drawn interest with the growing use of anticonvulsants in the treatment of bipolar disorder. These drugs enhance GABA transmission in the brain (Hardman, Limbird, & Goodman Gilman, 2001). In addition, bipolar patients, as compared with controls, show a marked reduction in the GABA-synthesizing enzyme, glutamic acid decarboxylase 65 and 67 messenger RNA in the hippocampus (Heckers et al., 2002).

Still, no one has yet articulated a comprehensive biochemical model that fully accounts for the initial onset of the illness, the appearance of manic and depressive episodes, and the effects of this broad array of pharmacologic agents. The signaling pathways mentioned earlier are undoubtedly involved in neuroplastic events that regulate complex psychological and cognitive processes, as well as diverse vegetative functions such as appetite and wakefulness. Consequently, in the clinical neuroscience community, considerable excitement has been generated by recent evidence that impairments of neuroplasticity and cellar resilience may underlie the pathophysiology of major depressive disorder, and that antidepressants and lithium exert effects on signaling pathways that regulate neuroplasticity and cell survival. Today, the best that can be said is that there is clearly a biochemical basis to bipolar disorder and we are moving closer to understanding the nature of the "chemical imbalance" associated with it.

Whatever the biochemical basis of bipolar I disorder, since the introduction of lithium in the 1960s, there has been an assumption that the disturbed biochemistry of this condition makes medication essential to its management. Unfortunately, it is only a minority of patients with bipolar disorder who can comfortably take the medications that seem to control the symptoms of the illness and who are willing to submit to this control. Especially early in the course of the illness, before it has wrought complete havoc in the patient's life, there is denial that there is anything permanently wrong and a longing for the highs that the medications take away. This makes treatment adherence an enormous problem in this patient population, a problem that every form of treatment must ultimately address if it is to be successful.

THEORIES RELATING TO CIRCADIAN DYSREGULATION

Another approach to understanding the physiologic basis of mood disorders in general, and bipolar disorder in particular, operates at the level of entire body systems and focuses on the role of the circadian system, or the body's "clock." Because theories of bipolar disorder relating to dysregulation of circadian systems figure so prominently in the rationale for the social rhythm aspects of IPSRT, it is important for you to be well informed about such theories in order to be able to present the strongest possible rationale for the treatment and to provide answers to questions that patients or their family members may have about the necessity of adopting regular routines. There is no question that the kinds of abnormalities in neurotransmission described earlier are associated with such circadian dysregulation; however, what is cause and what is effect, is not yet clear.

In their classic textbook on manic–depressive illness, Goodwin and Jamison (1990) argued that an integrated theory for understanding bipolar disorder can be based on an "instability model." Indeed, they "postulate that [instability] is the fundamental dysfunction in manic depressive illness" (p. 594).

For example, we saw in Jill's case how the combination of massive physiologic and psychosocial changes associated with the birth of a first child combined to lead to a first episode of illness in someone who, by leading a fairly orderly life prior to that point, had managed to avoid overt symptoms sufficient to qualify for a diagnosis of either depression or manic–depressive illness. In Tad's case, the precipitants appeared to be a combination of massive circadian disruption and intellectual and interpersonal over-stimulation.

A key component supporting the model proposed by our research group is derived from empirical data relating the sleep abnormalities observed in both depression and mania to the pathophysiology of the disorder. Our research group sought to place these sleep changes in the broader context of the pervasive circadian disturbances hypothesized in bipolar disorder. Finally, our work (Ehlers, Frank, et al., & Kupfer, 1988; Ehlers et al., 1993) has emphasized the relationship between psychosocial stressors (and, equally important, nonstressful alterations in the patterning of daily life) and changes in biological rhythms. Here, when we say "nonstressful," we mean not *psychologically* stressful in the conventional sense. However, many apparently benign (from a psychological standpoint) changes in daily routines can place considerable stress on the body's attempt to maintain synchronized sleep–wake, appetite, energy, and alertness rhythms.

Circadian rhythm researchers refer to the exogenous environmental factors that set the circadian clock as *zeitgebers* or "timegivers" (Aschoff, 1981). The primary and most powerful *zeitgeber* is the rising and setting of the sun, a physical *zeitgeber*. However, especially in urban, industrialized society, social factors such as the timing of work, meals, and even television programs have an important influence on circadian rhythms. We hypothesized that, in vulnerable individuals, changes in such social time cues may lead to disruptions in circadian rhythms and ultimately to affective episodes.

Biological theory holds that mood disorders are spontaneously occurring brain disease states produced by alterations in brain concentrations of neuropeptides, neurotransmitters, and/or neurophysiological and neuroendocrine abnormalities (Holsboer, 1995, 2000; Janowsky & Overstreet, 1995; Lewy, 1995; Maes & Meltzer, 1995; Modell, Ising, Holsboer, & Lauer, 2002; Nofzinger & Keshavan, 1995; Plotsky, Owens, & Nemeroff, 1995; Post et al., 1984; Riemann, Voderholzer, & Berger, 2002; Risch et al., 1984; Schatzberg & Schildkraut, 1995; Siever, Guttmacher, & Murphy, 1984; Thase, Frank, & Kupfer, 1985; Willner, 1995). More recently, this focus has shifted to the kinds of intracellular signaling pathways (e.g., Manji, Drevets, & Charney, 2001) mentioned earlier.

Although it may appear that multiple biological rhythm disturbances are present in mood disorders, there is no consensus as to whether a single underlying dysregulatory factor is responsible for the changes. For example, although rhythms of temperature and cortisol may be phase-advanced in depression (i.e., are shifted earlier in the 24-hour clock in depressed persons than in nondepressed individuals), the main feature of circadian rhythms during depression is the decreased amplitude of cortisol, thyroid-stimulating hormone, melatonin, and temperature rhythms, along with a change in their phase relationship (Sack, Rosenthal, Parry, & Wehr, 1987). Hypotheses exploring how disruptions in these important biological rhythms may occur have suggested that the "clock" or "clocks" that synchronize the phase relationships between sleep and other physiological functions, such as neuroendocrine rhythms, are malfunctioning (Wehr & Goodwin, 1983). How these clocks become disrupted in patients with mood disorders is still unclear; however, studies of the effect of light or day length suggest that light may play a role in the etiology and treatment of seasonal depressive disorders (James, Weh, Sack, Parry, & Rosenthal, 1985; Lewy, Sack, & Singer, 1985), possibly through its capacity to synchronize rhythms. Interestingly, studies in nonseasonal depression have not demonstrated that light is a primary synchronizing force in these patients' illnesses (Mendelson et al., 1986). Furthermore, the interaction of physical *zeitgebers* such as light with social *zeitgebers* has not been adequately explored, making it difficult to assess their respective roles in biological rhythm regulation.

PSYCHOLOGICAL AND PSYCHOSOCIAL THEORIES

To date, no one has articulated a purely psychosocial theory of bipolar illness itself; however, theories relating to effects of psychosocial factors on bipolar episodes and illness course are implicit in several of the psychological treatments described in Chapter 3. Most of these theories have not been described in any detail except in the treatment manuals for the respective interventions.

The various forms of psychoeducation described here grow out of an assumption that more knowledge about one's illness, about the medications used to treat it, and about how best to manage illness symptoms and medication side effects will lead to better treatment adherence, which will in turn lead to a more benign course of illness. These interventions also assume that patients and their families can be taught to recognize the early signs of impending episodes and that, having a well-defined plan of what to do when such signs are observed, may be able to prevent full syndromal relapse.

Manuals for the various cognitive therapies for bipolar disorder imply that the same patterns of dysfunctional thinking that are thought to be causal of unipolar depression are also relevant to bipolar depression. Some also theorize that just as patients can be taught to recognize and correct the irrationally *negative* thinking associated with depressive episodes, they can also be taught to recognize and correct the irrationally *positive* thinking associated with mania and hypomania. This is yet to be demonstrated empirically. Some of the cognitive therapies also acknowledge the (not always so irrational) negative cognitions bipolar patients have about their illness and about the medications they apparently must take to control it. Theoretically, if patients can modify these cognitions in a somewhat more positive direction, they may be better able to live with their disorder and better able to adhere to their medication regimens.

Ellicott, Hammen, Gitlin, Brown, and Jamison (1990) theorized that life stress, in the form of the kinds of negative life events already shown to be associated with the onset of unipolar depressions (Brown & Harris, 1979; Paykel & Tanner, 1976), was also relevant for the course of bipolar disorder. In studies conducted in the 1990s they demonstrated the temporal association between such events and relapse or recurrence of the disorder.

Brown and colleagues showed negative effects of a hostile family environment on the course of another psychotic disorder, schizophrenia, in the 1960s and 1970s (Brown, Birley, & Wing, 1972). This led to the development of a sophisticated system to measure "expressed emotion" (the presence of hostility, criticism, or emotional overinvolvement on the part of patients' parents or other family members) in the families of patients with schizophrenia (Vaughn & Leff, 1976). It also led to the development of family interventions based on the need to alter such environments to prevent relapse (Falloon et al., 1985; Hogarty et al., 1986).

Miklowitz, Goldstein, Neuchterlein, Snyder, and Mintz (1988) hypothesized that the same relationship between expressed emotion and relapse might apply to young patients with mania. In a longitudinal study of young adult patients recruited while hospitalized for a manic episode and returned to their families of origin, they demonstrated the relevance of such a negative family environment to the course of bipolar illness. Specifically, when parents expressed negativity toward patients in the form of highly expressed emotional attitudes, or when in face-to-face interactions with the patients, the patients were highly likely to relapse in the 9 months following hospitalization (94%). When family attitudes or interactional behaviors were benign, patients were much less likely to relapse (17%). Patients whose relatives showed negative interactional behaviors also showed lower social functioning at follow-up than patients whose relatives were benign in interactional behaviors. Similar associations between the emotional environment of the family and the course of bipolar disorder have been demonstrated in subsequent studies in the United States and Europe (Honig, Hofman, Rozendaal, & Dingemanns, 1997; Miklowitz et al., 2000; O'Connell, Mayo, Flatow, Cuthbertson, & O'Brien, 1991; Priebe, Wildgrube, & Muller-Oerlinghausen, 1989).

AN INTEGRATIVE THEORETICAL MODEL:
SOCIAL *ZEITGEBER* THEORY

In the late 1980s, we became increasingly dissatisfied with the "opposing camps" state of affairs in theorizing about the pathogenesis of mood disorders. Inasmuch as these illnesses were clearly occurring in individuals who showed evidence of both high levels of life stress *and* pathological entrainment of circadian rhythms (as well as other biological disturbances), we made an effort to integrate what was known about the biological basis of mood disorders with the strong evidence pointing to the role of stressful life events and absence of social supports in these illnesses. We proposed that specific social prompts (or social *zeitgebers*) be treated as unobservable variables that are inferred from the relationship between the occurrence of a life event and a change in the stability of social rhythms. Although the major hypotheses of the model are indicated by the cascading sequence shown in Figure 2.1, it is important to consider factors such as coping skills, social support, gender, and temperament as intervening variables within the model. In the primary path of the model there is a chain of events in which instability of social rhythms can lead to instability in specific biological rhythms, particularly sleep. The extent of instability is likely to be a function of the power of a particular relationship, task, or demand to set biological rhythms, that is, to act as a *zeitgeber*. The extent of instability and the appearance of consequent somatic symptoms are modulated by protective and vulnerability factors from both the psychosocial and the psychobiological spheres. These include the individual's coping skills, social supports, and temperament, as well as the flexibility of his or her particular biological clock. Such flexibility is exemplified by the individual's ability to adapt to a nighttime work shift, time zone changes associated with travel, or even the change from standard time to

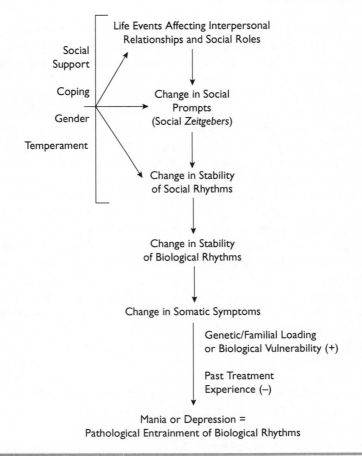

FIGURE 2.1. Schema for social *zeitgeber* theory.

daylight saving time and vice versa. We all know individuals who virtually never experience jet lag, who seem to have no trouble changing work shifts or even working a rotating shift, and who would laugh at the idea that the day we shift from standard to daylight saving time would have any impact on their mood or energy. We think of such individuals as having very "flexible" or adaptable biological clocks. We also know people who cannot adjust their work schedules by even a few hours or travel two time zones away without feeling awful. We think of those individuals as having "fragile" or inflexible biological clocks.

In vulnerable individuals (those with fragile clocks), the manic or depressive state then becomes the final psychobiological response to changes in the regularity of daily routines or social rhythms. In nonvulnerable individuals, biological rhythm disruption is self-limiting and is experienced only as mild somatic symptoms such as those observed under conditions of jet lag or, in some cases, as having no effect at all. In individuals vulnerable to mood disorder, however, the biological instability that leads to these somatic symptoms is not easily reversed but is potentially reversible. We believe that such individuals get stuck in a state of ongoing desynchronization or "pathological" entrainment of biological rhythms such as that observed in major depression and mania.

In our model, biological/genetic vulnerability factors exert the most powerful influence on whether biological rhythm instability actually leads to the alterations in biological rhythms that are often the hallmark of mood episodes, including shortened latency to REM sleep (Kupfer, 1978), abnormal cortisol levels and rhythms (Cassidy, Ritchie, & Carroll, 1998; Cervantes, Gelber, Kin, Nair, & Schwartz, 2001; Rush et al., 1996; Rybakowski & Twardowska, 1999) and altered sleep-associated growth hormone release (Mendelwicz et al., 1985). We believe that it is this disruption process that is often associated with the onset of the physical, cognitive, and affective symptoms that constitute the clinical criteria for an episode of mania or major depression. There is evidence to suggest that the biological changes associated with mood episodes, such as sleep abnormalities, may actually *precede* the reporting or observation of clinical symptoms of depression (Ehlers, Wall, Wyss, & Chaplin, 1988). According to our hypothesis, individuals at high risk for mood disorder, as a result of either a family history of affective disorder or a personal history of prior mood episodes, are more likely to move along the theoretical path illustrated in Figure 2.1 to the manic or depressed state that is its end point. Since the articulation of this hypothesis, our research group has conducted studies demonstrating that life events resulting in disruptions in such social routines are particularly salient predictors of the onset of manic episodes in individuals with bipolar disorder (Malkoff-Schwartz et al., 1998).

Once this biological rhythm disruption takes place, timing comes into play. When the individual "recovers" from the initial phase of the illness, his or her biological rhythms may return to normal; however, the risk of relapse or the onset of a new episode will depend on the relative balance of protective and vulnerability factors and on the presence or absence of rhythm-entraining social factors. It is for this reason that we emphasize the importance of social rhythm stability as one possible protective factor in individuals with a history of manic–depressive illness. Careful adherence to a mood-stabilizing medication such as lithium, valproate, or low-dose atypical antipsychotic is another important protective factor, but one that on its own may not be sufficient to protect vulnerable individuals from new episodes.

According to our model, the state of increased somatic symptoms that precedes depression or mania is a *normal* social and psychobiological response to a disruption in social rhythms and is usually self-limiting and reversible in nonvulnerable individuals. In fact, most individuals who develop the somatic symptoms associated with circadian disruption do not develop a major mood episode. The typical college student who "pulls an all-nighter" will feel a little off-kilter the next day, but will be feeling fine again the day after that.

Our theory also provides a framework for how both somatic and psychological treatment interventions serve to improve mood symptoms. Antidepressants have well-established direct effects on at least one biological rhythm (sleep) and probable effects on others (e.g., neuroendocrine and temperature rhythms) (Avery, Wildschiodtz, & Rafaelsen, 1982; Barden, Reul, & Holsboer, 1995; Goetze & Toelle, 1987; Golden et al., 2002; Leatherman et al., 1993; Soldatos & Bergiannaki, 2000). It may be that the biological changes produced by antidepressants can lead to changes in mood, concentration, and interest by setting the stage for circadian reentrainment. Much less is known about the circadian effects of the so-called mood stabilizer drugs (the list of which seems to be expanding monthly); however, some early studies did suggest that lithium had clear effects on sleep physiology (Kupfer, Reynolds, Weiss, & Foster, 1974)

In the same vein, it is of interest that two psychological treatment approaches that have been shown to be as efficacious as antidepressant medications in the treatment of major depression, Klerman and coworkers' interpersonal psychotherapy of depression (Klerman et al., 1984) and Beck and colleagues' cognitive therapy of depression (Beck, Rush, Shaw, & Emery, 1979), directly address at least one domain relevant to our hypothesis. Each of these complex and sophisticated short-term therapies focuses on different aspects of depression. Interpersonal psychotherapy (IPT) focuses on improving the quality and number of interpersonal relationships in the patient's life and on helping the patient to negotiate difficult transitions in social roles, whereas cognitive therapy attempts to alter his or her unrealistically negative cognitions. It should be noted, however, that in the process of improving the quality and number of social relationships or negotiating a role transition, IPT also serves to regulate daily and weekly social interaction. Perhaps even more directly relevant to our hypothesis, cognitive therapy usually begins with the attempt to establish regular daily routines of activity; only after such routines are established does intensive work begin on the patient's negative cognitive processes. Both of these effective therapies, then, serve to reestablish social *zeitgebers*.

SOCIAL *ZEITGEBERS* AND ENTRAINMENT OF CIRCADIAN RHYTHMS

The concept that social factors may synchronize circadian rhythms is not new (Wever, 1984). Indeed, until the late 1970s the vast majority of circadian rhythm research in humans concentrated on social cues, assuming that light–dark cycles played only a very minor role in setting human circadian rhythms in an urban society (Wever, 1988). Although since the 1980s there has been much more interest in the role of physical *zeitgebers*, it is still clear that social *zeitgebers* can be enormously potent as synchronizers of human circadian rhythms. For example, we know that when an individual is married, that individual tends to synchronize his or her rhythms to the rhythms of his or her marital partner. A couple's mealtimes, sleeping times, and times of activity and rest represent compromises between the two partners' natural individual rhythms. When a marital partner is lost through death or divorce, not only is there the emotional pain associated with that separation, but also the loss of a significant, if not primary, social *zeitgeber* (Hofer, 1984). The disruption of these social "regulators" is thought to have considerable effects on biological rhythms. The birth of an infant, who comes with his or her own highly intrusive rhythms, not only requires that the mother take on a new and demanding social role but also forces the mother and, to a lesser extent, the father to adapt their rhythms to those of the child. The loss of a job is also potentially associated with the loss of a potent *zeitgeber*, as well as the loss of an important source of self-esteem.

If the central physiological disturbance in mood disorders is a chronobiological one, events such as those described previously may have at least as much power to trigger mood episodes through the changes they precipitate in biological rhythms (particularly sleep rhythms) as through the psychological meaning of the events. In the 1980s, Cartwright (1983), demonstrated the biological impact of severely stressful events in a sample of divorcing community volunteers. More than half of a group of women going through divorce proceedings showed the shortened latency to REM sleep characteristic of the sleep of individuals with mood disorders as well as clinical evidence of depression.

ZEITGEBERS, ZEITSTÖRERS, AND AFFECTIVE ILLNESS

To account for the disrupting effects of life events that do not represent *losses*, we elaborated our *zeitgeber* theory, suggesting a new term, *zeitstörer*, or time disturber, to provide a further conceptual link between environmental changes, disruption of circadian rhythms, and affective disorders. The following paragraphs offer descriptions of some relevant social factors and how they might act as *zeitstörers* and thus possibly lead to affective illness in vulnerable individuals.

Transmeridian flight (flight across time zones) has been demonstrated to be a potent source, at least initially, of rhythm disruption. Circadian phase shifts induced by transmeridian flight have actually been shown to precipitate affective episodes, with the direction of flight predicting the prominence of manic versus depressive symptoms (Jauhar & Weller, 1982). Those flying east (particularly if they lose a night of sleep) are apt to become manic, whereas those flying west are more likely to become depressed.

Thus, transmeridian flight is a good example of a *zeitstörer*. When a person takes a transmeridian flight, he or she is exposed to new physical and social time cues (*zeitgebers*). Initially, this disrupts the person's rhythmicity. In nonvulnerable individuals, eventually these same time cues actually help to reset biological rhythms to be consonant with the new time zone. For example, when Klein and Wegmann (1974) restricted one group of transatlantic travelers to the confines of their destination hotel upon arrival, they suffered significantly more jet lag than those allowed to go "out and about."

Shift work represents a situation in which a *zeitstörer* can have a sustained effect, particularly for rotating shift workers, but also for permanent night shift workers who have daytime commitments when not working. Shift work exposes the individual to both physical and social factors that may be alternately entraining and disentraining their biological rhythms, depending on the time of day. It is not surprising that in addition to the jet lag-like symptoms of sleep disruption, malaise, and gastrointestinal disorders (Rutenfranz, Colquhoun, Knauth, & Ghata, 1977), shift work has been found to be associated with increases in divorce (Knutsson, Akerstedt, Jonsson, & Orth-Gomer, 1986; Tepas & Monk, 1987). Shift work is also associated with other maladies that may be related to the physiological challenges caused by circadian rhythm disturbance, such as increased risk of heart disease (Knutsson et al., 1986), difficulty concentrating and irritability (Rutenfranz et al., 1977), and heavier use of caffeine and alcohol (Gordon, Cleary, Parlan, & Czeisler, 1986). There appears to be a triad of factors—circadian rhythms, sleep, and social/domestic situations—that combine to determine a person's ability to cope with shift work (Monk, 1988; Regestein & Monk, 1991).

In our experience, individuals with mood disorders have a particularly difficult time with shift work. In some cases, the onset of the mood episode was directly associated with beginning shift work. In other cases, it seemed to interfere with the resolution of a depressive episode despite what is ordinarily effective treatment. This has often led us to indicate to employers that we consider this kind of work schedule incompatible with the patient's health and/or recovery and to request a change in his or her schedule.

Like a rotating shift schedule, a newborn baby in the home can lead to considerable sleep disruption, inconsistent bedtimes, inconsistent wake-up times, inconsistent exposure to sunlight, and inconsistent mealtimes. Indeed, the presence of a newborn can lead to an inability to plan or schedule virtually any aspect of the day and thus may act as a very potent *zeitstörer*. To our knowledge, no one has ever studied the relative vulnerability of mothers with calm, long-sleeping versus irritable, short-sleeping newborns to postpartum depressive episodes, but it would not be surprising if those in the latter group were more vulnerable to onsets of depression. In any case, the role transition of becoming a new parent not only provides many psychological and interpersonal challenges, it also represents a major challenge to the body's clock.

A hostile marriage can also act as a *zeitstörer*, as well as an emotional challenge. The fluctuation of emotional distress in either or both partners can lead to fluctuating periods of high emotional arousal, during which difficulty in falling asleep and loss of appetite can occur. More specific direct effects can occur as a result of open hostility that leads to inconsistent bedtimes, with marital partners going to sleep at more or less "regular" times when they are not arguing, but staying up much later or going to bed much earlier than usual when they are fighting with one another. Similarly, open hostility or a desire to avoid the partner can lead to inconsistent mealtimes as well as inconsistent composition of the family group at mealtimes. Finally, if the couple had ordinarily participated in a variety of leisure time activities together, the unavailability of one partner may lead to either a failure to participate in the activity or the choice of another time at which to carry out the activity. Some individuals seem able to tolerate the disrupting effects of such lifestyle changes. Others, particularly those with a history of mood disorder or sleep problems, may have considerable difficulty in tolerating this kind of social rhythm disruption.

In our social rhythm theory, we sought to integrate what was known at the time about the relationship between circadian rhythm changes in mood episodes with what was known about the relationship between life stress, especially interpersonal and social role stress, social supports, and the like, and onset of mood episodes into a single cohesive theory. It is based on the concept of *social zeitgebers*, those personal relationships, social demands, or more-or-less scheduled tasks that serve to entrain the biological rhythms discussed earlier in this chapter. Implicit in our theory was the idea that a treatment that could help patients to avoid or better manage challenges to their circadian system and help them to negotiate more stable, supportive social relationships and to prevent those stressful life events that depend partially on their own behavior, could ameliorate the course of recurrent mood disorders. And, indeed, that is what IPSRT appears to do.

SUMMARY

Bipolar disorder is a biologically based disorder in which multiple psychological and environmental factors play a strong role, especially in determining the course of illness and treatment response. Many theorists have remained focused in one realm or another. Instead, we have emphasized a theoretical perspective that attempts to integrate the apparently conflicting views of the illness, a perspective that forms the theoretical foundation for IPSRT.

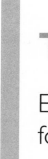

THREE

Empirically Supported Therapies for Bipolar Disorder

Before you can obtain your patient's commitment to participate in IPSRT, it is essential that you and your patient together evaluate the appropriateness of his or her pharmacotherapy regimen (perhaps in consultation with a psychopharmacologist if you are not yourself a physician) and that the two of you evaluate the appropriateness of IPSRT for this particular patient. To do this, you must be familiar with current approaches to the pharmacotherapy and psychotherapy of bipolar disorder. You must also be cognizant of what a key challenge pharmacotherapy adherence is in this patient population. Treatment adherence (or "compliance") is a challenge in all of medicine, but patients with bipolar disorder frequently have the additional problems of (1) denying that they have the disorder—What young person wants to believe that he or she has a psychotic illness that will last the rest of his or her life?—and (2) being told to take medications that actually take away the pleasant mild euphoria of hypomania and, instead, make the patients feel somewhat dulled and slowed down.

EMPIRICALLY SUPPORTED SOMATIC TREATMENT APPROACHES

Since the discovery and approval of lithium carbonate in the mid-20th century, pharmacotherapy has represented the mainstay of therapeutics for bipolar disorder. Indeed, initially the effects of lithium were seen to be so profound for this condition that research into other possible therapies came to a virtual standstill. In the initial trials of lithium, it appeared to have not only antimanic effects, but also antidepressant effects and long-term mood-stabilizing effects as well. It was perceived to be the "perfect" drug for bipolar disorder. In an era uncomplicated by the use of street drugs, outcomes for patients treated with lithium by its skilled and enthusiastic early proponents appeared to be outstanding. In the 1980s, however, reports of less than ideal outcomes with lithium began to appear. Both naturalistic studies of individuals being treated in the community (Harrow et al., 1990; Maj, Pirozzi, & Kemali, 1989; Markar & Mander,

1989; Tohen, Waternaux, & Tsuang, 1990) and controlled trials (Gelenberg et al., 1989; Potter & Prien, 1989) indicated that fewer than 50% of patients survived even 2 years without a new episode of illness.

Encouraged by the basic studies of Cutler and Post (1982) that suggested a kindling process similar to that seen in epilepsy might be responsible for the psychopathology of bipolar disorder, investigators began to explore the possible use of anticonvulsant medications for this condition. Although a sizable literature (Hlastala & Frank, 2000; Hlastala et al., 2000) has called the kindling theory into question, as a result of aggressive marketing by pharmaceutical companies anticonvulsant drugs have now come to supersede lithium as a treatment for bipolar disorder in many parts of the United States. The most commonly used of these is valproic acid or valproate (marketed as Depakote or Depakene). Depakote is approved for treatment of mania by the U.S. Food and Drug Administration (FDA); however, a number of other anticonvulsants that do not yet have FDA approval as treatments for bipolar disorder are also frequently employed for this purpose by clinicians in the United States and abroad. These include carbamazepine (marketed as Tegretol), which was actually the first of the anticonvulsants to be used in the treatment of bipolar disorder, and, more recently, topiramate (marketed as Topamax) and lamotrigine (marketed as Lamictal). Topiramate, although it does not appear to have profound symptomatic effects, may have the important benefit of reducing the weight gain associated with lithium, atypical antipsychotics, and other therapies for bipolar disorder and thus may constitute a viable adjunctive treatment. Lamotrigine has now been shown in at least two trials to have antidepressant effects in patients with bipolar disorder (Calabrese et al., 1999) and may also have some prophylactic effects against new bipolar episodes, especially new episodes of depression (Bowden et al., 2003; Calabrese et al., 2003)

There is now clear recognition that there are really a series of separate problems that need to be addressed in the pharmacotherapy of bipolar disorder: the treatment of acute mania; the treatment of acute depression, the treatment of acute psychosis (usually in the context of a mania, but sometimes also between full-blown episodes and sometimes in the context of depression), and the long-term prevention of future episodes of both mania and depression.

THE TREATMENT OF ACUTE MANIA

Acute mania is typically treated pharmacologically with large doses of a "mood stabilizer" such as lithium or valproic acid. If the mood stabilizer alone does not bring about a relatively rapid remission of manic symptomatology or if the patient is presenting with symptoms of psychosis, an antipsychotic medication is usually added to this treatment regimen. One of the clear goals of treatment of acute mania is sleep induction. Thus, antipsychotic and/or other sleep-inducing medication such as benzodiazepines will often be increased until several hours of continuous sleep are achieved. Although the older, typical antipsychotic drugs such as haloperidol (marketed as Haldol) or perfenazine (marketed as Trilafon) or even Mellaril are excellent for the purpose of reducing acute psychotic symptoms and inducing sleep, they carry a high side effect burden and risk of extrapyramidal side effects and even tardive dyskinesia with long-term use. Thus, the newer atypical antipsychotics, particularly risperidone (marketed as Risperdal) and olanzapine (marketed as Zyprexa), have be-gun to be used much more frequently in the treatment of bipolar disorder. Zyprexa was given a specific indication for the treatment of mania by the FDA in 2000. Tohen and colleagues (2002, 2003) have also now shown its prophylactic capacity in two well-designed controlled trials.

THE TREATMENT OF ACUTE BIPOLAR DEPRESSION

Although a subset of individuals with bipolar I disorder, perhaps 30–40%, presenting in an acute episode of bipolar depression respond to treatment with lithium or valproic acid alone, the majority do not. Indeed, many patients with bipolar disorder who pres-ent for treatment of an episode of depression are already taking a "mood stabilizer" that was ineffective in preventing their depressive episodes.

In patients with bipolar I disorder, antidepressant drugs are virtually always given only in combination with a mood stabilizer or an antipsychotic or both because of the fear of inducing mania. In patients with bipolar II disorder, however, antidepressants are frequently given alone. It may still be the case that the most efficacious treatments for bipolar depressions come from the class of drugs known as monoamine oxidase in-hibitors (MAOIs); however, they are rarely prescribed today because of both clinician and patient prejudice against them. This class of drugs includes tranylcypromine, mar-keted as Parnate, and phenelzine, marketed as Nardil (Himmelhoch, Thase, Mallinger, & Houck, 1991; Thase, Mallinger, McKnight, & Himmelhoch, 1992). The problem with the use of the MAOIs is the risk of hypertensive crisis when they are combined with certain foods or over-the-counter drugs. Inasmuch as the list of contraindicated foods includes things such as cheeses and other staples of today's fast-food diet, substantial numbers of patients, especially young patients, with bipolar disorder flatly refuse to take an MAOI. Because physicians are worried that patients who agree to take them may not be able to adhere to the dietary restrictions or may inadvertently eat a food or take an over-the-counter medication that interacts with the MAOI, they are often reluc-tant to prescribe them.

The older tricyclic antidepressant drugs, including amitriptyline, imipramine, and nortriptyline (marketed as Elavil, Tofranil, and Pamelor, respectively), have some anti-depressant effect in a subset of patients with bipolar illness. With these compounds, however, time to remission among patients with bipolar I disorder (perhaps because of the presence of a mood stabilizer) is often quite long and remission is often not nearly as complete as one would like it to be.

The newer antidepressants, particularly the SSRI drugs, are often used today in the treatment of bipolar depression and are appreciated for their somewhat less unpleasant side effects. Again, however, outcomes are often less than ideal. Time to remission in bi-polar I disorder is protracted and remission is often less than complete.

For a very long time the extraordinary difficulty of treating depressive episodes in the context of bipolar disorder was not explicitly discussed in the literature. The em-phasis was on the treatment of mania and on prophylaxis (mostly of mania) because this was what clinicians, patients, and family members worried about. This approach, however, left many bipolar patients to suffer protracted and debilitating (but not dra-matic) depressions. We now recognize that these low-grade depressions are actually associated with more impairment than the more dramatic, impressive manias (Judd et al., 2002), but this was not appreciated for much of the psychopharmacological drugs era.

More recently, Hlastala and colleagues (1997) and Kupfer and colleagues (2000) have pointed to the extraordinarily long times to stable remission of bipolar depressive episodes. The difficulty associated with the treatment of bipolar depression likely occurs because the antidepressant drug is almost always combined with a mood stabilizer that may, in fact, set limits on how "undepressed" (i.e., hypomanic) the individual can become.

MOOD STABILIZATION

As noted earlier, the ideal pharmacotherapy for bipolar disorder would bring depressed patients out of depression, manic patients out of mania, and prevent the return of either the depressive or manic symptomatology. In a subset of so-called classic bipolar patients, lithium does appear to have all of these properties. The early trials of lithium (Fieve, 1975; Gershon & Yuwiler, 1960; Schou, Juel-Nielsen, Stromgren, & Voldby, 1954) suggested long-term prophylactic effects against new episodes of illness; however, today's clinical experience with lithium maintenance is not nearly so positive as that reported in the years immediately following lithium's discovery. There are a number of hypotheses as to why this might be true. One thought is that this difference simply represents the typical disparity between early efficacy trials conducted in carefully selected patients at academic research centers by investigators who were passionate about the clinical care of those patients and convinced of the utility of the drug, and the "real-world" experience with more complex patients being treated by clinicians who are not necessarily specialists in the treatment of bipolar disorder. Another thought is that we have broadened our definition of what constitutes bipolar disorder in a way that includes many patients who do not have the "classic" features of those studied in the early lithium trials. A third hypothesis is that the population itself has become complicated by the broad availability of street drugs and the early onset of alcohol use, especially in those with a vulnerability to mood disorder.

More recently, clinicians searching for other options have begun to use valproic acid and the atypical antipsychotics as prophylactic agents in patients with bipolar disorder. In actual practice, bipolar patients who are not "lithium responsive" are often maintained on multiple medications including lithium, valproate, an antidepressant, and/or an antipsychotic in an effort to keep their mood stable. In a study examining a bipolar patient registry (Kupfer et al., 2002), we found that the typical patient was being maintained on four to five different medications.

What Is a Mood Stabilizer?

One of the confusing aspects of the pharmacotherapy of bipolar disorder is that there are three properties desirable in the ideal drug treatment for this condition. It should have antimanic effects in the case of an acute mania, antidepressant effects in the case of acute depression, and mood stabilizing or prophylactic effects in the long term. Indeed, when lithium was first marketed it appeared to have all three of these properties, and thus all future compounds were judged against this standard. First, it is no longer clear that lithium really does possess all of these properties to a significant degree in the majority of today's patients with bipolar disorder. It may still have all of these effects in a relatively small subset of patients with bipolar disorder, but the original "press" on lithium has clearly confused the picture when it comes to considering what really constitutes a "mood stabilizer." This confusion is enhanced by the fact that in order to receive an FDA indication for "bipolar disorder," drugs typically must first show their antimanic effect. Yet it may be that the ideal antimanic or antidepressant drugs in this population are not necessarily long-term mood stabilizing drugs. We appear to be on the threshold of a more rational approach to the approval of compounds for treatment of bipolar disorder in which each of the three properties of a drug will be evaluated separately. Still, the question of which drugs should be employed in which phases of the illness is not easily answered and a great many individual differences exist. If ever there was a patient population in which the clinician cannot be certain that the data on *average* effects will necessarily apply to an *individual* patient, it is this one.

Finally, there is the question of whether most of the currently employed mood stabilizers actually stabilize mood at a level that is in fact substantially below euthymia. It is our impression that in order to "keep a lid on" mania, many patients are "stabilized" in a state that might best be characterized as chronic mild depression. There may be instances in which this is a necessity, cases in which the severity and duration of mania has been so great and the damage done during manic episodes so profound that it is justifiable. We argue, however, that when the patient and clinician(s) have a good working alliance and are able to remain in reasonably close contact, the goal should be stabilization in a truly euthymic and fully functional state.

THE USE OF ANTIPSYCHOTIC MEDICATION IN THE TREATMENT OF BIPOLAR DISORDER

Although the most frequent use of antipsychotic medication has been for the acute treatment of mania, there was always a subset of patients with bipolar disorder who required low-dose antipsychotic medication on a prophylactic basis. These tend to be patients who experience more manias than depressions in the course of their bipolar disorder and patients in whom the complete discontinuation of all antipsychotic medication is associated with very rapid onset of hypomanic or manic symptomatology. As mentioned earlier, there is now good evidence that at least one of the newer atypical antipsychotic medications, olanzapine, has long-term prophylactic effects when used as a monotherapy (Tohen et al., 2002, 2003).

• *How many medications are needed to treat a patient with bipolar disorder?* Although monotherapy is considered the clear ideal in the treatment of *unipolar* depression, very substantial numbers of patients with bipolar disorder require polypharmacy in order to achieve anything that approximates stable mood and return to previous levels of functioning. It is a testament to the complexity and perniciousness of this disorder that a large minority, if not the majority, of individuals suffering from bipolar illness require complex medication regimens. For a fuller discussion of the pharmacotherapy of bipolar disorder and some of the currently suggested treatment algorithms, see the American Psychiatric Association Guideline for the Treatment of Bipolar Disorder and the report of the Texas Consensus Conference Panel on Medication Treatment of Bipolar Disorder 2000 (American Psychiatric Association, 2002; Goodwin, 2003; Suppes et al., 2002).

• *What stance should you take when a patient with bipolar disorder completely refuses to take medication?* As implied in the introduction to this chapter, complete refusal to take medication is not an uncommon problem in the treatment of patients with bipolar disorder, especially with those who are early in the course of their illness. Denial is a powerful coping mechanism and especially likely in the context of an illness in which one of the cardinal symptoms of the disorder itself is the patient's belief in his or her superiority and uniqueness.

In reality, each clinician has to make his or her own decision about what stance to take when a patient with bipolar I disorder completely refuses to take medication. Our approach, particularly with younger patients, has been to try to retain the connection with the patient, leaving the door open for the future addition of medication to the treatment regimen with the rationale that *some* connection to a well-informed clinician, who can remain alert to changes in symptoms and offer behavioral and psychological interventions that may mute symptoms, is better than no connection at all. We make it very clear at every possible opportunity that we think that psychotherapy alone is not an adequate treatment regimen for someone with bipolar I disorder, that we would feel more comfortable about the treatment were the patient taking medication, and that we hope that the patient will continue to consider the possibility of taking medication at some point in the future. Eventually, many of our patients have come to accept the idea of medication, usually when their mood has shifted from mild mania or hypomania to depression. However, we have seen cases in which the disorder was so severe and the potential for damage to self or others so great that we simply had to refuse to take clinical responsibility for the patient unless medicine were part of the treatment regimen.

For patients with bipolar II disorder or bipolar disorder NOS, psychotherapy alone may be a reasonable approach to both acute and maintenance treatment. Although we have not conducted an empirical study of IPSRT alone in this population, we have treated individual cases with good results. We have also had good outcomes with IPT alone in patients who would qualify for a diagnosis of bipolar II disorder.

EMPIRICALLY SUPPORTED PSYCHOSOCIAL AND PSYCHOTHERAPEUTIC TREATMENTS

• *Why add a psychosocial treatment to the pharmacotherapy of bipolar disorder?* With the recognition in the late 1980s (Coryell et al., 1993; Gitlin, Swendsen, Heller, & Hammen, 1995; Goodwin & Jamison, 1990) that outcomes even for those individuals with bipolar disorder who were well treated pharmacologically were less than ideal, came a renaissance of interest in the possible contribution of psychosocial treatments as adjuncts to pharmacotherapy in this population.

In the last decade of the 20th century, we recognized that psychotherapies that address the patient's psychosocial difficulties and enhance the patient's ability to manage the illness could play an important role in bridging the gap between symptom improvement brought about by medications and a full and sustained recovery (Potter &

Prien, 1989). Since that time, clinicians on both sides of the Atlantic have worked to develop a variety of individual, family, and group interventions to be used in combination with medication in the treatment of bipolar disorder.

The origins of these treatments are variable. Some, especially the psychoeducational approaches, came out of the simple recognition by psychopharmacologists who had no particular background in psychotherapy that their best efforts at providing appropriate pharmacotherapy were being frustrated by the notoriously poor treatment adherence among patients with bipolar disorder. They therefore set out to develop essentially atheoretical interventions aimed at improving pharmacotherapy adherence. Other interventions came out of clearly articulated theoretical models, mostly developed for disorders other than manic–depressive illness. Schizophrenia researchers, who had noted the negative effects of "expressed emotion" (i.e., hostility, criticism, and overinvolvement) in families of patients with schizophrenia, sought to apply their family intervention models to another psychotic illness, bipolar disorder. Psychotherapy researchers who had worked primarily with unipolar mood disorders sought to apply their models to bipolar patients and evolved individual treatment approaches based on cognitive or interpersonal therapy principles. As all of these treatments evolved and researchers began to discuss what they were *actually* doing in these treatments (as opposed to what they had originally conceptualized as the treatment protocol), it became apparent that there were certain common themes and treatment strategies that were being employed to a greater or lesser degree in all of them, strategies that form the basis of what is simply good clinical management of bipolar disorder.

As we approached the millennium, an ever-growing body of research indicated that, as compared with treatment with pharmacotherapy alone, treatment with the combination of medication and a bipolar-specific psychoeducational intervention or psychotherapy resulted in better outcomes for patients (Craighead, Milkowitz, Vajk, & Frank, 1998; Kusumakar et al., 1997; Swartz & Frank, 2001). Current treatment guidelines recommend the combination of psychotherapy with pharmacotherapy both for the acute treatment of bipolar depression and during the maintenance phase of the illness (American Psychiatric Association, 2002; Bauer et al., 1999; Frances, Kahn, Carpenter, Docherty, & Donovan, 1998; Yatham et al., 1997). Thus, psychotherapy now is considered an integral component of treatment for individuals suffering from bipolar disorder.

In general, the treatment guidelines and consensus documents recommend mood stabilizer pharmacotherapy as a first-line treatment for bipolar depression, followed by the addition of either psychotherapy or antidepressant medication. Interestingly, in most of these documents psychotherapy is marginally favored over antidepressant medication as a primary augmentation strategy, probably because of concern that antidepressant medication could induce mania whereas psychotherapy is thought to be unlikely to do so. For the treatment of a nonpsychotic depressive episode, the 1998 U.S.-based Expert Consensus Guidelines (Frances et al., 1998) recommends initiating or optimizing a mood stabilizer before adding one or more of the following interventions: (1) a specific psychotherapy, (2) an antidepressant medication, and (3) electroconvulsive therapy (ECT) (p. 21). This group noted that at that time psychotherapies had not been well studied in bipolar depression, but argued that psychotherapy is likely to be of benefit especially when the depressive episode seems to have been precipitated or exacerbated by psychosocial stressors (p. 16). Since then, several groups have published results indicating the positive effects of psychotherapy on bipolar depression, and these are described in detail in the following paragraphs. The U.S. Department of Veteran Affairs' Guideline (Bauer et al., 1999) for the treatment of bipolar disorder made recommendations similar to those of the Frances and colleagues work group. The Veteran Affairs (VA) module for depression, however, *begins* with an "evaluation for on-going psychotherapy and/or psychosocial rehabilitation" at the same time that mood stabilizers are initiated or optimized (Bauer et al., 1999, p. 15) and explicitly recommends that antidepressant medication be used conservatively. A Canadian work group focusing on the treatment of bipolar depression (Yatham et al., 1997, p. 88) suggests optimizing existing mood stabilizer treatment before adding a second mood stabilizer, an antidepressant, or psychotherapy; however, this may not reflect actual practice. In a survey of 766 Canadian psychiatrists, 84% of respondents said they would combine psychotherapy with somatic interventions as their first-line treatment approach for bipolar depression (Sharma, Mazmanian, Persad, & Kueneman, 1997).

• *What kinds of empirically supported psychotherapies are available for bipolar disorder?* Today, many psychosocial approaches to the treatment of bipolar disorder are described in the literature. They include individual, family, and group psychoeducation; group therapy; couple therapy; family therapy; individual interpersonal psychotherapy; and individual cognitive-behavioral therapy. However, for many of these treatments there is as yet relatively little in the way of empirical evidence of efficacy. Your obligation, in introducing and obtaining your patient's agreement to participate in IPSRT, is to present reasonable alternatives to IPSRT. It is important that you know about other treatments that have been shown to be helpful and can describe them in a general way to your patient. The American Psychological Association's (APA) convention for labeling a treatment as "empirically supported" has been the existence of two adequately powered positive controlled studies (Crits-Cristoph, Frank, Chambless, Brody, & Karp, 1995), although other kinds of evidence such as data from carefully designed mirror-image studies are also important to consider in a developing area like this one. At this point, no treatment for bipolar disorder meets the APA standard, with the possible exception of family-focused treatment (FFT) developed by Miklowitz and Goldstein. FFT has been shown in separate sizable studies conducted in Los Angeles and in the Denver/Boulder, Colorado, area to prevent relapse and rehospitalization and diminish ongoing depressive symptomatology (Miklowitz et al., 2000; Rea et al., 2003).

What is even more problematic is that, of the treatments that have shown some evidence of efficacy, very few have published treatment manuals or established therapist-training procedures. Other treatments have been well described in lengthy published treatment manuals, but have not been tested empirically. Furthermore, the few clinicians trained in the apparently efficacious treatments are found almost exclusively at academic medical centers. In other words, although alternatives to IPSRT clearly exist, it may be very difficult for your patient to find competent clinicians trained to provide these treatments.

As noted earlier, the empirically supported psychotherapies for bipolar disorder have tended to come from one or two arenas: (1) empirically supported treatments for other psychotic disorders such as schizophrenia and (2) empirically supported treatments for unipolar disorder. Those clinical researchers who had had experience working primarily with psychotic disorders tended to focus on the psychoeducational family and marital interventions that had been successful in preventing relapse and rehospitalization in patients with schizophrenia, and those who had worked with unipolar mood disorders tended to focus on individual treatments.

We describe in the following sections only those treatments for which there is at least some evidence of efficacy, either in the form of controlled data or a well-designed mirror-image study in which carefully collected data on pretreatment course are compared with posttreatment course. We have categorized the treatments described by their apparent operational technique; however, as noted earlier, there is considerable overlap among these therapies and the categorization may sometimes seem arbitrary. Table 3.1 provides a summary of the evidence supporting the approaches discussed here.

Psychoeducation (Group and Individual)

Colom, Vieta, and their colleagues in Barcelona, Spain, have developed a group psychoeducational intervention for euthymic patients that consists of 20 90-minute sessions focused on the illness. The treatment addresses four main issues: (1) illness awareness, (2) treatment compliance, (3) early detection of prodromal symptoms and recurrences, and (4) lifestyle regularity. In the last two sessions some attention is also given to problem solving and stress management. Patients who received this structured educational intervention had significantly longer survival time without a new episode of illness; however, even in those who received the intervention there was about a 60% probability of recurrence over the subsequent 2 years (Colom et al., 2003).

Investigators from the University of Manchester (United Kingdom) have shown that a brief (7- to 12-session) individual cognitive-behavioral psychoeducational intervention may be useful in preventing manic relapses. The intervention is designed to help euthymic patients identify the early symptoms of relapse. The typical patient received only nine hour-long individual sessions conducted by a relatively inexperienced clinician. The treatment focused on helping subjects to identify their particular prodromal patterns (for both mania and depression) and outline a plan for action if the prodromal symptoms emerged. The therapist recorded the specific plans on laminated cards, which the subjects carried with them at all times. Patients who received this intervention demonstrated significantly longer time to first manic relapse, but there was no difference in time to first depressive relapse. There was also a significant reduction in the total number of manic relapses over 18 months, but no difference in the total number of depressive relapses. Thus, an individualized relapse prevention strategy appears to be able to decrease the frequency of manic recurrences over a 1½-year period.

Group Therapy

Bauer and McBride (1996) have developed the Life Goals Program, a structured group therapy program that employs psychoeducational, cognitive-behavioral, and interpersonal strategies to diminish symptoms and overcome social and occupational limitations for patients being treated for bipolar disorder through the U.S. Veterans Administration. Phase I consists of five highly structured psychoeducation sessions that provide information about the illness, its treatment, and early warning signs of relapse. Phase II is an open-ended, more flexible group in which a patient identifies at least one social,

TABLE 3.1. Psychosocial Treatments for Bipolar Disorder

Lead investigators (year)	Psychotherapy modality	No. of subjects (comparison of subjects)	Mean duration of treatment	Major outcome(s)	Comments
Basco & Rush (2005)	Individual (cognitive-behavioral)	0 (0)	20 sessions	Unspecified	Manualized treatment, but not yet tested
Cerbone et al. (1992)	Group (psychodynamic and psychoeducation)	43 (0)	1 year	Decreased hospitalization	Retrospective chart review
Clarkin et al. (1990)	Family (psychoeducation)	12 (9)	8.6 sessions	Improved global functioning	Inpatient intervention
Clarkin et al. (1998)	Marital (psychoeducation)	18 (15)	11 months	Improved overall functioning and improved medication adherence	
Cochran (1984)	Individual (cognitive-behavioral)	14 (14)	6 weeks	Lower rates of lithium noncompliance	
Colom et al. (2003)	Group (psychoeducation)	60 (60)	2 years	Reduced number of relapsed patients, number of recurrences per patient, and longer survival time without a new episode	
Davenport et al. (1977)	Marital group	12 (53)	1 year	Decreased hospitalization and improved social functioning	
Glick et al. (1991)	Individual and family (psychoeducation)	24 (0)	Unspecified	Resolution of acute episode better with psychoeducation	Retrospective, cross-national study
Graves (1993)	Group (supportive)	14 (0)	2.9 years	Decreased hospitalization	
Jacobs (1982)	Individual (cognitive)	0 (0)	2–4 years	Unspecified	Treatment for "dysphoria"
Kripke & Robinson (1985)	Group (supportive)	17 (0)	10 years	Decreased hospitalization and improved socioeconomic function	
Lam et al. (1999, 2003)	Individual (cognitive-behavioral)	51 (52)	20 sessions	Reduction in relapse, higher medication blood levels, improved social functioning	

Study	Treatment type	N (control)	Duration	Outcome	Comments
Miklowitz et al. (2000, 2003)	Family (psychoeducation)	31 (70)	9 months	Improved rate of relapse-free survival; decrease in depressive symptoms	Largest trial in the series
Palmer et al. (1995)	Group (cognitive-behavioral)	4 (0)	17 sessions	Improved well-being	
Peet & Harvey (1991)	Individual (psychoeducation)	30 (30)	2 sessions	Improved lithium knowledge	
Perry et al. (1999)	Individual (psychoeducation)	34 (35)	7–12 sessions	Increased time to manic relapse; decreased number of manic relapses; no effect on time to depressive relapse	Maintenance study; subjects followed for 18 months
Rea et al. (2003)	Family (psychoeducation)	28 (25)	21 sessions over 9 months	Reduced risk of relapse or rehospitalization	Same intervention as used in the Miklowitz et al. studies
Scott et al. (2001)	Individual (cognitive-behavioral)	21 (21)	25 sessions over 6 months	Improved symptoms and functioning; decreased relapse rate	
Simon et al. (2003, 2005)	Group (psychoeducation, cognitive-behavioral, and interpersonal)	0 (0)	5 sessions (phase 1) plus open-ended treatment (phase 2)	Improved knowledge, functional status, symptom severity, quality of life, illness costs	
Van Gent et al. (1998)	Group (psychoeducation)	20 (14)	10 sessions	75% of patients (vs. 29% of controls) "improved" (self-report)	
Van Gent & Zwart (1991, 1994)	Group (psychoeducation)	14 (12)	5 sessions	No change in patient adherence to medications	Group for patients' partners
Volkmar et al. (1981)	Group (interpersonal and "interactional")	20 (0)	47 sessions	Improved lithium levels and decreased hospitalization	
Wulsin et al. (1988)	Group (psychodynamic)	22 (0)	44 sessions	Unspecified	
Zaretsky et al. (1999)	Individual (cognitive-behavioral)	11 (11)	20 sessions	Reduction in depressive symptoms	Matched-case control design; unipolar depressed control subjects

37

occupational, or leisure goal that has been disrupted by bipolar disorder. Examples of goals identified in the manual include having a safe pregnancy without experiencing illness symptoms, not missing work while depressed, and getting a job. Using worksheets, the group member and therapist develop a graded behavioral strategy to attain the goal. An effectiveness study of the Life Goals Program, conducted in a large health maintenance organization, found that a systematic care program for bipolar disorder significantly reduced risk of mania over 12 months. Results suggested a growing effect on depression over time, but indicated that a longer follow-up period would be required (Simon, Ludman, Unutzer, & Bauer, 2002; Simon et al., 2005).

Cognitive-Behavioral Therapy

Not surprisingly, the individual therapy that has received the most development and research attention for bipolar disorder is that which has received the most research attention for unipolar disorder: cognitive therapy. Several groups in North America, the United Kingdom, and elsewhere have developed various adaptations of Beck's (Beck et al., 1979) cognitive therapy for the treatment of patients with bipolar disorder. Common elements among all of these cognitive therapies include a cognitive approach to medication adherence, a cognitive-behavioral approach to symptoms of depression that includes both the behavioral interventions (increasing activity and increasing experiences leading to a sense of mastery or pleasure) and the correction of negative thinking that are characteristic of Beck's cognitive therapy. Efforts are also made in some of these treatments to "correct" the cognitive distortions associated with hypomania/mania; however, it is not yet clear that this can actually be done. Basco and Rush (2005) published a detailed treatment manual for a cognitive therapy of bipolar disorder, but this version of the treatment has not, to our knowledge, been tested empirically.

Several other groups have developed unpublished manuals for cognitive-behavioral therapy for bipolar disorder (Lam, Jones, Hayward, & Bright, 1999; Lam et al., 2002; Newman, Leahy, Beck, Reilly-Harrington, & Gyulai, 2001; Otto, Reilly-Harrington, & Sachs, 2003; Scott, Garland, & Moorhead, 2001), but only two had published outcome data at the time of this writing. Lam and colleagues (1999, 2002) describe an acute treatment (20 sessions) that emphasizes the identification and management of prodromal symptoms and the discussion of long-term issues such as stigma, shame, and loss, in addition to a focus on psychoeducation, treatment adherence, and symptom monitoring. The treatment of the depressive phase of the disorder relies on standard cognitive-behavioral techniques such as challenging negative automatic thoughts, cognitive reframing, graded task assignment, and problem solving. Their version of the treatment was associated with significant reduction in rates of relapse, improved medication adherence, and improved psychosocial functioning, as well as significantly fewer days in a bipolar episode and fewer hospital admissions.

The cognitive-behavioral model of Scott and colleagues (2001) involves four primary elements: (1) socialization into the cognitive-behavioral model and development of an individualized formulation and treatment goals, (2) cognitive and behavioral approaches to symptom management and dysfunctional thoughts, (3) dealing with cognitive and behavioral barriers to treatment adherence and modifying maladaptive beliefs, and (4) anti-relapse techniques and belief modification. According to their model, socialization into cognitive-behavioral therapy involves exploring the patient's understanding of the disorder, a discussion of previous episodes, a careful review of prodromal signs, both the clinician and the patient obtaining some understanding of the stressors associated with onsets, and an exploration of the patient's interpersonal functioning. The cognitive-behavioral approaches to symptom management involve the teaching of self-monitoring and self-regulation techniques and exploring skills for coping with depression and mania, including regular activity in the establishment of daily routines, methods for coping with stress, use of time management and social support, and then addressing dysfunctional thoughts. What may be a unique feature of the Scott and colleagues approach is the extent to which the treatment addresses barriers to treatment adherence through exploration of what those barriers might be and through a challenging of automatic thoughts related to medications, to bipolar disorder, and to self-reliance. This, of course, leads to the use of cognitive and behavioral techniques aimed at increasing adherence to treatment. Finally, the treatment involves a series of antirelapse techniques including the recognition of early signs of relapse, the self-monitoring of symptoms so that such early signs are apparent, the development of a list of risk situations, and a clear plan for how to cope after the termination of cognitive-behavioral treatment. The treatment consisted of 25 sessions over 6 months. In an initial study, at 6-month follow-up, subjects who received cognitive-behavioral therapy showed statistically significantly greater improvements in symptoms and functioning than those in a waiting-list control group. Relapse rates in the 18 months after commencing cognitive-behavioral therapy showed a 60% reduction in comparison with the 18 months prior to commencing therapy. Scott and colleagues noted that although the results of this study are encouraging, the use of cognitive-behavioral therapy in subjects with bipolar disorders is more complex than among those with unipolar disorders and requires a high level of therapist expertise. Scott and colleagues have now conducted a large multisite trial of their version of cognitive-behavioral therapy; however, results from this investigation had not been published at the time of this writing.

Marital and Family Therapy

Several groups have studied marital and family interventions for patients with bipolar I disorder. Clarkin, Glick, and colleagues (Clarkin et al., 1990; Clarkin, Haas, & Glick, 1988; Glick, Clarkin, Haas, Spencer, & Chen, 1991; Haas et al., 1988; Spencer et al., 1988) developed an inpatient family intervention (IFI) and tested this intervention in groups of hospitalized patients that included some individuals with bipolar disorder. IFI encourages patients and family members (1) to accept the reality and chronicity of the disorder and the fact that both medical and psychosocial treatment will likely be necessary following hospital discharge, (2) to identify stressors both within and outside the family that may be related to the onset of psychiatric episodes, and (3) to learn ways to modify family patterns and to cope with future episodes and stressors. They compared their treatment to hospital treatment alone in a large controlled trial ($N = 186$) of hospitalized patients with a variety of disorders and found treatment effects were strongest for female patients with mood disorders (including bipolar disorder) both at hospital discharge and at 6- and 18-month follow-up. Effects were seen mostly on attitudinal measures rather than on symptomatology.

Clarkin, Carpenter, Hull, Wilner, and Glick (1998) have also described a psychoeducational marital intervention for bipolar outpatients and their spouses. This intervention had a three-part focus: (1) improving spousal communication and attitudes, (2) educating the marital partners about the disorder, and (3) enhancing adherence to pharmacotherapy. Patients enrolled in the marital treatment demonstrated significantly higher overall functioning and medication adherence as compared with those receiving medication management alone. There were no differences in levels of symptomatology between the two groups; however, this study suggests the possible value of a marital intervention for those patients with bipolar disorder who are married.

The most carefully studied family intervention is the 9-month family psychoeducational treatment developed by Miklowitz and Goldstein (1997). Family-focused treatment (FFT) is delivered in 21 sessions over a period of 9 months and consists of three modules: (1) a psychoeducational intervention offering information about bipolar disorder and how to cope with bipolar symptomatology, (2) communication enhancement training, and (3) problem-solving skills training. Results from an initial pilot study (Miklowitz & Goldstein, 1990) and two subsequent randomized trials (Miklowitz et al., 2000; Rea et al., 2003;) have all indicated significant effects for this very focused intervention. FFT was associated with greater probability of survival without a relapse into a syndromal episode and longer survival times during the first year. In addition, FFT appears to reduce ongoing depressive, but not necessarily manic/hypomanic symptomatology in this population.

IPSRT

The efficacy of IPSRT has been examined in two controlled studies. The first investigation, conducted at the University of Pittsburgh, compared IPSRT plus manual-driven pharmacotherapy with an intensive clinical management (ICM) paradigm plus manual-driven pharmacotherapy as acute and maintenance treatments in patients with bipolar I disorder. The same nonphysician clinicians provided either IPSRT or ICM, depending on the patient's randomization. The ICM condition consisted of 10 elements, including (1) education about bipolar disorder, (2) education about the medications used to treat bipolar disorder, (3) detailed inquiry about symptoms, (4) detailed inquiry about any possible medication side effects or somatic symptoms, (5) medical and behavioral management of side effects/somatic symptoms, (6) education about basic sleep hygiene, (7) identification of and strategies for management of early warning signs of impending episodes, (8) use of rescue medication where indicated for impending episodes, (9) nonspecific support, and (10) the availability of a 24-hour on-call service.

In our research group's initial study, 175 acutely ill patients with bipolar I disorder were randomly assigned to one of four psychosocial treatment strategies: acute and maintenance IPSRT, acute and maintenance ICM, acute IPSRT followed by maintenance ICM, or acute ICM followed by maintenance IPSRT. The preventative maintenance phase lasted 2 years. As mentioned earlier, all study participants received protocol-driven pharmacotherapy. We were interested in whether IPSRT would reduce the time required to reach stabilization in the acute treatment phase and whether it would increase survival time without a new episode in the preventative maintenance phase. We defined stabilization as 4 consecutive weeks over the course of which the subject's Hamilton Rating Scale for Depression scores and Bech–Rafaelsen Mania Rating Scale scores each averaged ≤7, or, in other words, a practically symptom-free state. Recurrence was defined as meeting criteria for a new major depressive, manic, or mixed episode. We were also interested in whether the treatment strategies would differ with respect to the amount of mood symptomatology and instability experienced between episodes during the 2-year maintenance phase. We hypothesized that IPSRT would be associated with shorter time to stabilization, longer time survival time without a new episode, and greater affective stability than ICM.

What we found was somewhat different from what we had expected. IPSRT did not differ from ICM in terms of the speed with which subjects reached a stable, essentially symptom-free state; however, it turned out that those subjects who received IPSRT in the *acute treatment phase* survived significantly longer without a new affective episode during the 2-year *maintenance phase*, and this was true whether they continued to receive IPSRT in the maintenance phase or not. Furthermore, among those subjects who were treated acutely with IPSRT, their ability to increase the regularity of daily routines during the acute treatment phase was associated with significantly reduced likelihood of recurrence during the subsequent 2 years. Average levels of mood symptomatology over the course of maintenance treatment were low for all subjects and did not differ among the four randomized treatment conditions. IPSRT appeared to be particularly efficacious for those subjects with relatively good medical health and those without a history of lifetime anxiety disorder. For subjects with high levels of medical burden and a history of lifetime anxiety disorders, the more somatically focused ICM appeared to be a better treatment option. We concluded that treatment with IPSRT following an acute bipolar episode that is sustained until the patient has fully stabilized typically has a protective effect against new episodes of illness. For the majority of the patients we treated in our study we did not see any additional benefit to continuing the treatment beyond the point of full stabilization; however, it should be remembered that the individuals we studied were essentially symptom-free at that point and were generally adherent to their medication regimens. Patients who are struggling with these issues or who are still trying to achieve stable routines or interpersonal relationships may benefit from further treatment with IPSRT.

Our results suggest that the best time to initiate IPSRT is when a patient is either acutely ill (for depressive episodes) or just beginning to recover (for manic or mixed episodes). This seems to be the time when patients are most motivated to make the kinds of lifestyle changes that IPSRT typically requires. We found no evidence that beginning IPSRT when a patient has been stable for a long time is in any way harmful; however, for fully stable patients, doing so did not appear to confer any extra protective effect against new episodes. If the goal of treatment of a symptomatically stable patient, however, is resolution of interpersonal distress or negotiation of a difficult role transition, starting IPSRT in a stable individual may make a great deal of sense.

IPSRT is also being studied in the large multicenter Systematic Treatment Enhancement Program for Bipolar Disorder (STEP-BD) sponsored by the National Institute of Mental Health. In this investigation it is being compared with cognitive therapy, FFT, and a control condition known as Collaborative Care Plus (CC Plus). Final results from the psychosocial treatment arm of STEP-BD are not likely to be published until 2006. Some early analyses did, however, suggest that IPSRT was associated with significantly better treatment adherence than the other psychosocial treatments.

In presenting the rationale for IPSRT to your patient, you can describe the empirical support for the treatment itself and for the theories that underpin it, as well as the evidence that the psychoeducational components of the treatment have been shown in multiple studies to be beneficial to patients with bipolar disorder. You might also mention the substantial empirical evidence that the interpersonal components represent efficacious acute and maintenance treatments for unipolar disorder.

FINAL THOUGHTS

As a clinician working with patients with bipolar disorder, you have several key responsibilities at the time you initiate IPSRT: (1) to ensure, to the extent possible given your own clinical competencies and the patient's ability to access treatment, that the pharmacotherapy the patient is receiving is appropriate to his or her current clinical condition and history of illness; (2) to ensure that the patient is well informed about the medications he or she is taking; (3) to ensure, to the extent possible given the patient's current living circumstances and social network, that close family members and/or significant others have sufficient information about the illness to be able to provide reasonable support to the patient; and (4) to have achieved a reasonable degree of certainty, based on a discussion of the patient's needs and the nature of other empirically supported therapies available to the patient, that IPSRT represents an appropriate intervention at this time. A full discussion with your patients and their family members or significant others about all the reasonable treatment options available can aid greatly in discharging these responsibilities and in gaining your patient's commitment to the treatment enterprise ahead.

FOUR

A Brief Overview of Interpersonal and Social Rhythm Therapy

Interpersonal and social rhythm therapy is essentially a prophylactic treatment for a chronically recurring disorder. The goal of therapy is primarily to prevent new episodes of illness or, at least, to extend the interval between episodes. According to our model, there are likely to be three paths to new episodes of illness in bipolar patients maintained on lithium carbonate or other mood stabilizers: (1) nonadherence to medication; (2) stressful life events, especially interpersonal events and changes in social roles; and (3) disruptions in social rhythms. IPSRT specifically addresses each of these potential pathways. By providing a forum in which patients can explore their feelings about having the disorder, grieve for what we have called "the lost healthy self," and come to terms with how the disorder has altered their lives, IPSRT attempts to reduce denial and increase acceptance of the lifelong nature of the illness and its never-to-be-underestimated propensity to recur. This tends to have a powerful positive effect on medication adherence. By addressing interpersonal problems and social role transitions, IPSRT attempts to reduce the number and severity of interpersonally based stressors patients experience and the impact of such stressors both on patients' mood and, indirectly, on the regularity of their social routines. Finally, IPSRT focuses careful attention directly on the regularity of patients' daily routines (both the timing of events and the amount of stimulation they produce) with the goal of directly increasing the regularity of patients' routines and their vigilance with respect to maintaining that regularity.

We see the reduction of interpersonal stress in this patient population as being important for several reasons. First, stressful life events can have a direct effect on circadian integrity through increased autonomic arousal leading to reductions in sleep and appetite. Second, many stressful (and not so stressful) life events lead to marked changes in daily routines. Even a small thing like a child's moving from elementary to middle school and needing to be at the bus stop an hour earlier can prove very challenging to the circadian system of someone with bipolar disorder. Third, truly stressful events, like losing one's job or getting divorced, not only lead to marked changes in social routines, but also typically have a direct and negative effect on mood, leaving the patient vulnerable to a new episode of depression.

THE BASIC ELEMENTS OF IPSRT

The basic elements of IPSRT, like those of its predecessor, IPT, are the management of affective symptoms and the resolution of interpersonal problems. When offered as an acute treatment, the goals of IPSRT are the improvement of the affective symptoms and the resolution of the interpersonal problem(s) most closely linked to the onset of the most recent affective episode. When used as a prophylactic maintenance treatment, the goals are to maintain a euthymic mood state and to improve (and prevent any new crises in) the patient's interpersonal life and social role functioning.

Management of Affective Symptoms

For patients with bipolar I disorder, the management of affective symptoms is accomplished through the use of appropriate pharmacotherapy and through efforts to regularize their social rhythms. For patients with bipolar II disorder, depending on the severity of the mood symptoms, IPSRT may be offered either as a stand-alone intervention or along with pharmacotherapy. In either case, stabilizing social rhythms is a key aspect of the management of mood symptoms.

Resolution of Interpersonal Problems

Resolution of the patient's interpersonal difficulties and maintenance of good interpersonal and social role functioning is accomplished by selecting from the interpersonal problem areas specified by Klerman and colleagues (Klerman et al., 1984; Weissman et al., 2000). IPT defines four key problems areas: unresolved grief, social role transitions, interpersonal role disputes (usually with a spouse, parent, or child), and more generalized interpersonal deficits (chronic isolation or chronic dissatisfaction with most or all interpersonal relationships). In IPSRT we added a fifth problem area that we call "grief for the lost healthy self," which refers to the sense of disconnection from the prediagnosis self that many individuals with bipolar I disorder feel. In addressing these problem areas, we use largely the same strategies and tactics as those employed in IPT for unipolar patients. These are described in detail in Chapter 9.

THE INITIAL TREATMENT PHASE

Whenever possible (i.e., assuming the patient is not in crisis), the initial phase of treatment should begin with a focused *history taking*, intended to develop the rationale for the treatment, by emphasizing the extent to which disruptions in social routines and interpersonal problems or social role transitions have been associated with affective episodes. This is true whether the patient is first seen in an acute episode or in a period of remission. Also in this initial phase, you will provide the patient (and his or her family, when indicated) with *education* about his or her mood disorder, taking into consideration what the patient has already learned or not learned about bipolar illness. You will *assess the quality of your patient's interpersonal relationships* through a process known as the Interpersonal Inventory, described in detail in Chapter 6. You will also *assess the regularity of your patient's social routines* by asking him or her to complete the Social Rhythm Metric, a monitoring device also described in detail in Chapters 6 and 7. Finally, you and your patient will *select an interpersonal problem area* (the one that will become the initial focus of therapy) from the five IPSRT problem areas (unresolved grief, role transitions, interpersonal role disputes, interpersonal deficits, or grief for the lost healthy self. This initial phase of treatment typically lasts three to five sessions, depending on the length and complexity of the patient's affective history, the complexity of his or her interpersonal relationships, and the amount of psychoeducation required.

Obviously, if the patient first presents for treatment (or is assigned or brought to you) in an acute manic episode or in an acute crisis, this sort of orderly approach to treatment is not possible.

If your first contact with your patient occurs when he or she is in a manic psychosis (and presumably in the hospital), the most you may be able to do is establish an interpersonal connection and wait for the medication to take its course. During that time it will, nonetheless, be important to have regular contact, perhaps even daily if possible, to make clear your level of concern and interest. Even wildly psychotic individuals can perceive concern and empathy and, indeed, may be hypersensitive to such behavior of the clinician.

If the patient is too manic to proceed with an orderly history taking, but not psychotic, you may first provide a general overview of what will happen in the treatment once he or she is a bit more stable, and explain the general philosophy of the treatment. You should try to ensure that the patient is receiving appropriate pharmacotherapy and adhering to the prescribed medication regimen. If adherence seems to be a problem, you may want to select the IPSRT intervention modules aimed at improving adherence and employ them to the extent possible, given the patient's clinical status. If overstimulation seems to be contributing to the mania or preventing the full resolution of the episode, you can attempt to discuss this with the patient. All of your attempts to intervene at this point, however, may well be frustrated by the patient's lack of insight and desire to remain in what may feel to him or her like a very pleasant, productive, exciting state. If this is the case, you may be limited to attempts to point out the potentially negative consequences of the mania. If your patient lacks insight and is irritable and argumentative, it may require all your clinical skills just to maintain a connection until the mania resolves.

If the first clinical contact occurs in the midst of an acute interpersonal or vocational crisis, as is often the case with this population, our approach has been to focus almost exclusively on the crisis. The following is a step-by-step description of our approach:

- Ask the patient to describe the nature of the crisis.
- Let the patient talk.
- Limit your interventions. Just letting the patient talk or cry may be enough to calm him or her down.

- Listen, show interest. This may be enough to establish a relationship. Do not try to talk about issues that are not strictly pertinent to the crisis, unless the patient introduces those issues him- or herself. This will avoid irritating the patient or giving the patient the impression that you do not understand or care about what is going on in his or her life.
- Evaluate whether it is safe to treat the patient on an outpatient basis.
- Discuss the factors that may have contributed to the crisis.
- Ask the patient to describe what is happening right now with respect to the crisis.
- Discuss what the factors are that are continuing to contribute to the crisis. What is sustaining the current situation? This inquiry is likely to give you a basic idea of the patient's interpersonal issues and a preliminary idea of the level of disruption of the patient's rhythms.
- Ask the patient to describe what he or she thinks will happen.
- Discuss what the factors are that may make the crisis worse.
- Reevaluate whether it is safe to treat the patient on an outpatient basis.
- Discuss what the factors are that may improve the current situation.
- Provide the patient with an emergency plan in case the situation becomes much worse.
- Describe the goals of the treatment that you plan to provide, and give the patient an idea of how the sessions will be organized.
- Arrange for another visit with the patient within 3–5 days.

THE INTERMEDIATE PHASE OF TREATMENT

Once you have concluded the initial phase of treatment, you will move on to the intermediate phase of therapy. In this phase, you focus on *regularizing the patient's social rhythms* and *intervening in the selected interpersonal problem area*. A full chapter is devoted to each of these two goals later in this book. Chapter 8 focuses on social rhythm regularity, and Chapter 9 describes the strategies and tactics for intervening in each of the interpersonal problem areas.

Typically, IPSRT is provided weekly in the initial and intermediate phases, but other schedules may be appropriate if the patient is either very symptomatic, in which case more frequent visits may be needed, or fully remitted and in treatment primarily to try to improve current functioning and prevent future episodes. For such patients, once a good alliance is established, biweekly or monthly visits may be more appropriate for this intermediate phase of treatment.

THE CONTINUATION OR MAINTENANCE PHASE

The continuation or maintenance phase of IPSRT is the phase in which you will work to establish patients' confidence in their ability to use the techniques learned earlier in the treatment. These include *maintaining regular social rhythms*, even in the face of challenges such as vacations, job changes, and unexpected life disruptions, and *maintaining or further improving their interpersonal relationships*. Specific techniques for accomplishing these goals are also outlined in Chapters 8 and 9. As the treatment moves from the intermediate to the continuation or maintenance phase, the frequency of visits is typically reduced from weekly to bimonthly and, eventually, to monthly.

THE FINAL PHASE OF TREATMENT

The final phase of IPSRT may involve work toward *termination of therapy* or further *reduction in the frequency of visits*. When termination is seen as an appropriate goal or is necessitated by financial concerns or a move, this is usually accomplished over the course of three to five monthly visits. Alternatively, the final phase of treatment may involve a further reduction in the frequency of visits to something more like occasional check-ups or booster sessions. Given the apparently lifelong nature of bipolar illness, this is probably the preferred option whenever continued contact is possible. In our experience, even patients who have done very well in acute and maintenance IPSRT benefit from being able to check in with their therapists every 3–4 months simply to review how things are going. This approach has proven to be particularly helpful when a patient has become ill again. The intervening contact makes it much easier to reinstitute therapy, because the therapeutic relationship has remained intact and the therapist is familiar with the current state of the patient's interpersonal world.

In some cases it may be necessary or preferable to offer only an acute course of IPSRT, lasting 16–20 sessions, in which the emphasis is on education and resolution of the acute mood episode. When the contract is for short-term treatment, the initial phase of treatment may need to be compressed and work on the interpersonal problem area very focused. When this is the case, our experience with briefer forms of IPT for unipolar depression (see Swartz et al., 2004) suggests that you are well advised to focus on the accomplishment of a single obtainable goal in the interpersonal arena. For example, if your patient has been engaged in a long-standing marital dispute that is unlikely to be resolved without months of work, you might choose instead to focus on your patient's "transition" to a more satisfying social or volunteer life that is not dependent on resolving the conflicts in the marriage. There may even be instances of short-term treatment with IPSRT in which virtually all of your time is spent on efforts to stabilize your patient's social rhythms, with relatively little time spent focusing on a specific interpersonal problem area. Even when IPSRT is provided as a short-term treatment, it is probably advisable to reduce the frequency of the sessions toward the end, allowing for three to four biweekly sessions during which the termination work is accomplished.

USING A MODULAR TREATMENT APPROACH

In some respects, IPSRT can be thought of as a series of treatment modules (an assessment module, a psychoeducation module, a social rhythm regularization module, and several interpersonal problem area modules) that can be employed and reemployed throughout a course of treatment. Which modules you will use and when will depend on the patient's affective state at the time he or she enters treatment and what happens in the patient's life over the course of treatment. These modules, in turn, are all nested in a context of supportive clinical management (see the sections on medication monitoring and side-effect management in Chapter 10) that may be considered still another module upon which the clinician draws on a regular basis.

We initially designed IPSRT for intervention for a randomized controlled study of acutely ill patients who, once their acute symptomatology had remitted, were then followed for 2 years of maintenance treatment. Because of the design of that study, however, one fourth of our subjects did not begin IPSRT until their acute episodes were fully remitted. In the process of conducting the study, we found that IPSRT can be begun either when patients are acutely ill or in a state of remission. In subsequent chapters we describe a chronology of IPSRT treatment modules that grew out of this experience; however, many other approaches to IPSRT are possible and the specific difficulties being experienced by specific patients may suggest alternate sequencing of the various modules described in this book. For example, we tended to incorporate most of the education about the disorder into the history-taking process, but there were certainly times when we returned to the education module later in the treatment. If the patient experienced a new episode of the polarity opposite to the one that brought him or her to treatment in the first place, that was often an occasion for additional education. Likewise, if a patient became involved in a new relationship or reengaged in an old one, we might offer the option of a conjoint psychoeducational session at whatever point in treatment it seemed appropriate.

Often, we put considerable emphasis on social rhythm stabilization early in treatment. Once a patient had established fairly regular routines, we just did a quick review of the Social Rhythm Metric on a regular basis to be sure that the regularity was being maintained, but did not spend much time on this module of the treatment. We did work hard to weave "social rhythm talk" into our interpersonal interventions, but did not do active *intervention* to alter social rhythms unless events in the patient's life seemed likely to pull against his or her established routine and direct intervention seemed necessary to maintain stability.

IPSRT is relatively easy to implement in motivated patients who have accepted their illness as a fact of their lives. The patient who is still in partial denial about the power of bipolar disorder or its lifelong nature represents more of a challenge for the IPSRT clinician. For such patients, moving quickly to work on grief for the lost healthy self, and thus targeting the denial that so frequently stands in the way of treatment adherence and good outcome for patients with bipolar disorder, is often a good idea.

Although we typically select one interpersonal problem area to focus on in the beginning of treatment, other interpersonal problem foci might well prove appropriate later in the therapy, particularly if the patient's circumstances have changed. Moreover, as we discuss in detail in Chapter 9, sometimes the interpersonal problem area most closely linked to the onset of the patient's episode (e.g., a marital role dispute), is too threatening as an initial focus of treatment and focusing on it directly runs the risk of early termination. In that case, we try to find an alternate focus that is acceptable to the patient with which to begin the therapy, and hope to return to the more salient but more threatening problem area when the patient feels better and the therapeutic alliance is stronger. In other cases, new interpersonal or social role problems arise *during* treatment (e.g., a change in the patient's job responsibilities), particularly if the treatment is in the maintenance phase. When this occurs, we make use of the role transition module of the treatment, generally adapting it to the less frequent contact of the maintenance phase, but possibly scheduling a few more closely spaced visits at the time of the role change.

IPSRT is intended to allow considerable flexibility to use those modules of the intervention package that seem most appropriate to the patient's clinical state and interpersonal circumstances at various times during treatment. Thinking of the various parts of the treatment as modules that can be taken off the shelf when needed can be very helpful in enabling you to individualize the therapy. What is important is to be certain that each patient is given adequate exposure to each of the key components at some point during the treatment.

FIVE

Assessment of Bipolar Disorders and Common Comorbidities

Before you can decide whether IPSRT is the right treatment for any individual patient, you must first decide whether he or she has a bipolar disorder. This is best accomplished through a systematic, structured diagnostic assessment. When such an assessment is done with a presumption that a course of IPSRT will follow, we tend to weave a good deal of psychoeducation into the diagnostic process. (More about how to do that is provided later in this chapter.)

Given the dramatic nature of its symptomatology, it may seem that the diagnosis of bipolar disorder should be a very straightforward matter, but this is often not the case. A number of factors can complicate the process of obtaining an accurate diagnosis. First, in almost all cases, the diagnosis of bipolar disorder is essentially a longitudinal rather than cross-sectional one. Although it is true that according to DSM-IV (American Psychiatric Association, 1994), a single episode of mania qualifies an individual for a diagnosis of bipolar I disorder, the illness usually presents first as depression sometime in adolescence or early adulthood. Sometimes these depressive episodes are severe enough to come to clinical attention, but more frequently they are written off by both the young person and those around him or her as adolescent moodiness or a "bad semester." Further complicating the picture is the fact that first episodes of mania, when they are severe and psychotic, may be indistinguishable from a first episode of schizophrenia. Such episodes are often brief (too brief for the clinicians involved to get a full picture of the symptomatology) and since return to prior functioning is often complete, the patient sees the episode as some odd aberration rather than part of the evolving longitudinal clinical picture that it actually represents. Indeed, in a patient registry of individuals with bipolar disorder, we found that typical registry participants spent a decade between the time they experienced their first symptoms and the time they received a correct diagnosis (Kupfer et al., 2002). A survey of members of the Depression and Bipolar Support Alliance (formerly the National Depressive and Manic–Depressive Association) provided similar data. Still, unless a patient is overtly psychotic or unwilling or unable (because of lack of insight or denial) to cooperate, the clinician who can take the time to obtain a careful history of mood symptoms and episodes should be able to make the diagnosis of bipolar I disorder accurately.

When expanded to include the diagnosis of bipolar II disorder (episodes of depression alternating with episodes of *hypomania*), the diagnostic workup can be very challenging. Hypomania is, by definition, a much more subtle condition than mania, and many factors can serve to obscure its presence. First, many individuals who suffer from bipolar II disorder can see their episodes of depression as distinct from their "normal selves," but find their hypomanic periods more consistent with their normal temperament. Second, hypomania is a highly desirable state in most instances, because the sufferer experiences high levels of energy, interest, enthusiasm, and productivity. Any implication on the part of the clinician that this is a disorder may be met by disdain or disbelief or both, causing patients to be less than fully forthcoming about their experiences. Third, because a key criterion for the diagnosis is that the change in behavior be observable to others, without reports from family members or significant others it may be difficult to determine what the patient's normal baseline is and what represents a deviation.

All that being said, the essential feature of an episode of depression consists of sad or empty mood associated with clear changes in neurovegetative functioning, including sleep, appetite, and weight; changes in cognitive functioning, including the ability to concentrate and remember; and changes in interest and energy. These are often accompanied by marked reductions in self-esteem, pessimism, unrealistic guilt, and thoughts of death or suicide. Depressed mood or loss of interest in usual activities must be present, along with at least four of the other criterion symptoms most of the day for a period of at least 2 weeks; although in practice, individuals with bipolar depression often suffer for many months before seeking clinical attention.

In contrast, the essential feature of mania is an episode of 3 days or more of high, irritable, or expansive mood accompanied by an unrealistically high self-esteem; neurovegetative changes, including decreased appetite and need for sleep; high energy and interest; poor judgment; and a tendency to become involved in behaviors with a high risk for negative social consequences, including reckless driving, overspending, sexual promiscuity, and the like. These symptoms are often accompanied by racing thoughts, which may not be apparent to the clinician, and rapid or disorganized speech, easily recognized by others. In order to qualify for diagnosis, these symptoms must lead to impairment, as evidenced by problems in work, social and/or family functioning, trouble with legal authorities, or behavior that could have led to such trouble if detected (e.g., reckless driving that does not lead to arrest). In its more severe forms, mania involves delusional thinking, usually focused on the individual's capabilities and/or on religious or spirituality themes, although paranoia and delusions of persecution may also be present.

Complicating both the immediate and longitudinal diagnosis of mania and hypomania is the tendency for patients to normalize relatively outrageous behaviors both for the clinician and in their own eyes. Often a clear picture can be obtained only by meeting with significant others or other outside observers of the patient's behavior.

As implied earlier, hypomania can be the much more difficult clinical state to identify. The criteria for an episode of hypomania require a more sustained period characterized by many of the essential features of mania (expansive or irritable mood, high energy, lack of need for sleep, etc.) without any evidence of the impairment in functioning that is a requirement for the diagnosis of mania. A final problem complicating the recognition and diagnosis of manic/hypomanic states is the subtle continuum from normal energy and enthusiasm, through the kind of hypomania that is observable to others but not really dysfunctional, to manic behavior that is clearly impairing and even psychotic. Even very experienced clinicians seeing a patient on a regular basis can miss the early stages of mania, particularly when the symptoms come on very gradually and are consistent with the patient's normal enthusiasms and interests. Indeed, in such instances frequent contact may make the upward swing in mood more difficult to detect.

Bipolar disorder can also present in the form of a so-called mixed episode, often referred to as a "mixed state." The strict DSM requirement for a mixed episode is the *simultaneous* presence of a sufficient number of criterion manic *and* criterion depressive symptoms to qualify for both diagnoses. Mixed states that meet these stringent criteria are relatively rare, at least in outpatient settings. Many patients with bipolar disorder, however, present a somewhat more subtle mixed picture. Indeed, some experts on bipolar disorder adhere to the belief that all bipolar episodes are mixed: Even in the most severe bipolar depression, one occasionally sees transient evidence of manic or hypomanic features, and even in the most severe mania one often sees a very sad, dysphoric facial expression and other evidence of dysphoria when the patient is caught in repose.

An important aid in the establishment of a presumptive diagnosis of bipolar disorder when the diagnostic picture is not entirely clear is the family history of mood disorders. Of all the mood disorders, bipolar disorder appears to have the strongest genetic component. Thus, it is very useful to know about the presence of manic–depressive illness (as well as any hospitalizations for severe depression, psychosis, "nervous breakdowns") in both first- and second-degree relatives of the patient. The probability that a bipolar diagnosis is the correct one in a young individual whose symptom picture has not fully clarified increases dramatically when the family history is characterized by the presence of clear-cut bipolar I disorder.

As noted earlier, the true diagnosis of bipolar disorder is made on a longitudinal basis, except in those rare conditions when a patient presents in a clear-cut episode of mania not preceded by any history of depression. Thus, your task involves an emphasis on the history of mood episodes, as well as on the presenting complaint. In our experience, patients often come to clinical attention in a first episode of mania sometime in their early 20s, denying that they have ever experienced an episode of depression. Indeed, their depressions may not have been identified at the time. When you have an opportunity to educate the patient about what depression looks like in adolescence (characterized by a good deal of irritability, overeating, and oversleeping, rather than by the more typical symptoms of melancholic depressions) and then review the patient's adolescence semester-by-semester and summer-by-summer, you can often find extended periods of presumptive depression, marked by uncharacteristically poor academic and social functioning.

Further complicating the diagnostic process and the presentation of the diagnosis to patients and families is the fact that, relative to other mood disorders, bipolar disorder or manic–depressive illness is a much more highly stigmatized condition. This is generally not a diagnosis that patients want to receive, nor is it a diagnosis that family members want them to have unless they have spent years suffering from the symptoms without appropriate treatment or hope of relief. In such instances, it can actually be reassuring to learn that this is a condition that is well known to medical science and for which there are proven treatments.

EDUCATING PATIENTS (AND FAMILY MEMBERS) ABOUT BIPOLAR DISORDER

As noted earlier, when diagnostic assessment is done in preparation for IPSRT, we tend to weave the assessment together with patient and family education about the disorder.

Individuals who come for treatment of their manic–depressive illness appear with widely varying amounts of knowledge about their condition. Some have had years of good treatment, have been directed to accurate information by well-informed and caring clinicians, and have read everything they could find that seemed legitimate. Others, despite years of treatment for the disorder, have been told essentially nothing by those treating them, except to take their medication, and have tried in vain to learn about their condition from the vast array of popular books and magazine articles, websites, and other unvetted sources. Still others, who have managed to survive years of illness in a supportive (and often enabling) family environment without receiving formal treatment, know nothing about the disease and are ambivalent at best about learning more about a condition they are not at all convinced they actually have. Finally, and most challenging of all, are the young patients who have just experienced their first psychotic episode and do not want to learn anything at all about a condition they are certain they do not have. Yet essential to the management of this chronic disease is finding a way to educate each of these patients about their condition.

The well-informed patient should be asked about his or her specific beliefs about the condition and then corrected if any misperceptions exist. Sometimes a good history of the patient's illness will reveal that these are not, in fact, misperceptions, but rather, correct observations that patient has made about atypical aspects of his or her own disorder. For example, although epidemiological data suggest that women with bipolar disorder are likely to experience more episodes of depression than mania in their lifetimes, some women actually have the opposite experience. Such patients will need to be much more on guard for impending mania than depression. Moreover, conventional wisdom may suggest (and most reading material will state) that few patients taking only lithium can be effectively protected against new episodes of illness if their lithium levels are below 0.6 mEq/liter; however, we have certainly seen exceptions to this generally sound advice.

The patient who presents having read widely, but with little guidance or selectivity, may have many idiosyncratic ideas about his or her illness. Again, the IPSRT disease management strategy begins with trying to achieve an understanding of exactly what the patient has come to believe about manic–depressive illness. Has he bought the notion that all manic-depressive patients are either creative geniuses or business phenoms and is left wondering why he has been such a failure? Does she believe what her church has told her, that even a disease as serious as this one can be overcome without treatment if only she becomes strong enough in her faith? Has he been told that the "real thing" is always treatable with mood stabilizers alone and that if he needs a neuroleptic as well to maintain stability, he must have schizoaffective disorder or some other form of schizophrenia? Once you have a clear picture of the patient's knowledge and beliefs, you can decide whether you are the best person to address each part (e.g., history, symptoms, medications, side effects, etc.) of the education of the patient. If you are providing both the patient's pharmacotherapy and psychotherapy, then obviously all of this work devolves to you. If the patient has a physician who is providing pharmacotherapy, he or she may be the best person to educate the patient about medications and their side effects.

DIFFERENTIAL DIAGNOSIS

Bipolar disorder presents two kinds of differential diagnosis problems, both of which can be helped by conducting the kind of structured diagnostic interview discussed in the following paragraphs. The first challenge is to determine whether the patient actually has bipolar disorder, a different disorder, or both bipolar disorder and one of the disorders that can sometimes be difficult to separate from bipolar disorder.

When an exited, psychotic patient presents in an emergency or inpatient setting, the differential diagnosis is most often between mania and schizophrenia, schizoaffective disorder, or acute psychosis. Unless the patient is accompanied by a relative or friend, it may be very difficult to obtain the kind of historical information necessary to determine whether this episode is part of a bipolar picture. Indeed, many patients who in the end prove to have bipolar disorder are misdiagnosed at first hospitalization simply because, without the longitudinal picture, the differential diagnosis may be difficult if not impossible.

When patients present on an outpatient basis, the two conditions that are most likely to be confused with bipolar disorder are borderline personality disorder and, in younger patients, attention-deficit/hyperactivity disorder (ADHD). Borderline personality disorder overlaps in many respects with bipolar disorder, including the presence of labile mood, irritability, impulsivity, and instability of social relations. ADHD overlaps in some respects with bipolar disorder as it presents in childhood, especially in terms of hyperactivity and impulsivity. Further complicating the differential diagnosis problem is that both borderline personality disorder and ADHD can also be comorbid with true bipolar disorder.

Differentiating bipolar disorder from borderline personality disorder can be a challenge for even the most experienced clinician. As Table 5.1 illustrates, many of the criterion symptoms for the two conditions simply represent the same behaviors or internal experiences called by different names. The picture becomes even more confusing when the bipolar disorder is of the rapid-cycling form. Assuming it is not, the cardinal features distinguishing the two conditions are discrete and usually long periods of low mood accompanied by the vegetative changes of major depression, or periods of truly elated mood accompanied by the poor judgment of mania (for bipolar disorder) and desperate efforts to prevent abandonment or parasuicidal behavior (for borderline personality).

In children and adolescents, distinguishing bipolar disorder from ADHD can be an equally difficult task. Again, the problem of symptom overlap complicates the differential diagnosis. As Table 5.2 indicates, the criterion symptoms of mania (elation, no need for sleep, inappropriate sexual behavior) can be important guides, as can a family history of bipolar disorder. Although IPSRT has been developed for adults and older ado-

TABLE 5.1. **Symptoms of Bipolar Disorder and Borderline Personality Disorder**

Symptom	Bipolar	Both	Borderline
Depressed mood		×	
Irritable mood		×	
A distinct period of abnormally and persistently elevated or expansive mood		×	
Affective instability due to a marked reactivity of mood (e.g., intense episodic dysphoria, irritability, or anxiety usually lasting a few hours and only rarely more than a few days)			×
Markedly diminished interest or pleasure in all, or almost all, activities	×		
Inflated self-esteem	×		
Low self-esteem		×	
Identity disturbance: markedly and persistently unstable self-image or sense of self			×
Significant weight loss when not dieting (e.g., a change of more than 5% of body weight in a month)	×		
Significant weight gain (e.g., a change of more than 5% of body weight in a month)	×		
Decrease in appetite	×		
Increase in appetite	×		
Grandiosity	×		
Chronic feelings of emptiness			×
Insomnia		×	
Hypersomnia	×		
Decreased need for sleep (e.g., feels rested after only 3 hours of sleep)	×		
Excessive involvement in pleasurable activities that have a high potential for painful consequences (e.g., engaging in unrestrained buying sprees, sexual indiscretions, or foolish business investments)		×	
Impulsivity in at least two areas that are potentially self-damaging (e.g., spending, sex, substance abuse, reckless driving, binge eating)		×	
Psychomotor agitation (observable by others, not merely subjective feelings of restlessness)		×	
Psychomotor retardation (observable by others, not merely subjective feelings of being slowed down)	×		
More talkative than usual	×		
Pressure to keep talking	×		
Inappropriate, intense anger		×	
Difficulty controlling anger (e.g., frequent displays of temper, constant anger, recurrent physical fights)		×	
Fatigue		×	
Loss of energy		×	

(continued)

TABLE 5.1. (continued)

Symptom	Bipolar	Both	Borderline
Flight of ideas	×		
Subjective experience that thoughts are racing	×		
Transient, stress-related paranoid ideation		×	
Severe dissociative symptoms			×
Feelings of worthlessness		×	
Excessive or inappropriate guilt (which may be delusional and which is not merely self-reproach or guilt about being sick)	×		
Feelings of hopelessness		×	
Distractibility (i.e., attention too easily drawn to unimportant or irrelevant external stimuli)	×		
Frantic efforts to avoid real or imagined abandonment			×
Diminished ability to think or concentrate		×	
Indecisiveness		×	
Increase in goal-directed activity (socially, at work or school, or sexually)	×		
A pattern of unstable and intense interpersonal relationships characterized by alternating between extremes of idealization and devaluation		×	
Recurrent thoughts of death (not just fear of dying)	×		
Recurrent suicidal ideation without a specific plan		×	
A specific plan for committing suicide		×	
A suicide attempt		×	
Recurrent suicidal threats, gestures, or behavior			×
Self-mutilating behavior			×

TABLE 5.2. **Tips to Differentiate Bipolar Disorder from Attention-Deficit/ Hyperactivity Disorder**

Suspect the presence of bipolar disorder in a child with ADHD if:

- The symptoms of ADHD appeared later in life (e.g., at 10 years old or older).
- The symptoms of ADHD appeared abruptly in an otherwise healthy child.
- The symptoms of ADHD were responding to stimulants and now are not.
- The symptoms of ADHD come and go and tend to occur with mood changes.
- A child with ADHD begins to have periods of exaggerated elation, depression, no need for sleep, inappropriate sexual behaviors.
- A child with ADHD has severe mood swings, temper outbursts, or rages.
- A child with ADHD has hallucinations or delusions.
- A child with ADHD has a strong family history of bipolar disorder, particularly if the child is not responding to appropriate treatments.

Remember that an individual may have *both* ADHD *and* bipolar disorder.

Note. From Birmaher (2004). Copyright 2004 by Three Rivers Press. Adapted by permission.

lescents, making it unlikely that you will be seeing children in the context of providing IPSRT, knowing about the ADHD differential diagnosis will be important in your history taking and, at times, in helping your patients to understand what is happening with their children.

The differential diagnosis between schizoaffective and bipolar disorders is made on the basis of interepisode psychosis. In other words, if patients continue to have delusions or hallucinations when their episodes of mania or depression are fully resolved, they are considered to have schizoaffective disorder. Sometimes this is quite obvious, making the differential diagnosis an easy one. At other times, the patient's interepisode suspiciousness or ideas of persecution may have sufficient basis in reality that it is difficult to determine whether they actually represent delusional thinking.

Finally, it is important to think about the differential diagnosis with recurrent unipolar disorder. In our experience, many patients with bipolar disorder spend years, often as much as a decade, being treated for unipolar depression before receiving a correct diagnosis. This is especially likely to happen to individuals with bipolar II disorder and those with bipolar I disorder whose manias are nonpsychotic.

Among all the differentials discussed here, the questions that are really important for you to consider from an intervention standpoint as an IPSRT therapist are whether these differentials might affect your decision to use IPSRT in the first place and, if so, what the prognosis might be. We have used IPSRT with good success with patients who have both bipolar disorder and borderline personality disorder (Swartz, 2005; Swartz et al., 2000); however, the time course to full mood stability was much longer for these patients, about a year in most cases, than in patients who had only bipolar disorder. We have no experience using IPSRT in individuals who qualify only for a diagnosis of borderline personality disorder, although Angus and Gillies (1994) have reported using IPT successfully in the treatment of depression in patients with borderline disorder. More recently, Markowitz and colleagues (in press) have written about possible mechanisms of change in patients with borderline personality disorder treated with IPT.

As to patients with schizoaffective disorder, we included patients with a schizoaffective manic diagnosis in our IPSRT trial and did not find that they were necessarily less responsive. This differential is important primarily because it has implications for the patient's pharmacotherapy. These are individuals who will almost always require antipsychotic medication as part of their long-term treatment regimen.

SUBTYPES OF BIPOLAR DISORDER

The second challenge is differential diagnosis among various forms of bipolar disorder, defined in DSM-IV as bipolar I disorder, bipolar II disorder, cyclothymic disorder, and bipolar disorder not otherwise specified (NOS). Unlike the therapeutic approach in unipolar disorder, in which the initial treatment for multiple forms (i.e., major depressive episode, minor depressive episode, chronic depression, or dysthymia) is likely to be the initiation of one of the depression-specific psychotherapies or an SSRI, the differences between the various forms of bipolar disorder have substantial treatment relevance. Pharmacotherapeutic treatments that are entirely appropriate for the patient with bipolar I disorder may not be appropriate for the patient with bipolar II disorder or bipolar disorder NOS, especially in their milder forms, and almost certainly are not appropriate for those with cyclothymia. Likewise, treatments that are appropriate for patients with bipolar II disorder or bipolar disorder NOS may be inadequate to control the symptoms of bipolar I disorder. The distinction between bipolar I and II disorders is made on the basis of the presence of mania versus hypomania, but this distinction is often one that turns on whether the episode meets the *impairment* criterion required for mania. In actual practice, this can be a difficult distinction to make. For example, the man who buys 12 new sweaters on a single day, and can easily afford all 12 and more, does not meet the impairment criterion, whereas the man who buys 12 but clearly cannot afford even one new sweater meets the criterion. The young woman who reports regularly speeding on the country roads near her home, but is never caught, does not meet the criterion, but the young woman who gets three speeding tickets in a week meets that criterion.

Fortunately, with respect to the decision of whether to initiate IPSRT, we believe it is an appropriate intervention for patients with bipolar I and II disorders and probably for many patients with bipolar disorder NOS. As the patient's IPSRT clinician, what you will want to be cognizant of as you prescribe, or consult with a prescribing physician, is which form of bipolar disorder your patient has. You will also want to know whether your patient has comorbid conditions that may affect his or her response to various pharmacotherapy regimens or to IPSRT itself.

METHODS FOR OBTAINING A DIAGNOSIS OF BIPOLAR DISORDER

Probably the most common method for obtaining a diagnosis of bipolar disorder is an unstructured interview in which the diagnostic requirements for depression and mania or hypomania, according to the DSM, are reviewed. In the hands of a clinician who is fully familiar with the extended descriptions provided in the DSM (as opposed to just the summary lists of criterion symptoms), such an interview can be an appropriate diagnostic tool; however, studies of the extent to which even well-trained clinicians succeed in making correct diagnoses on the basis of unstructured interviews point to the clear benefits of validated structured interviews (Shear, Greeno, et al., 2000; Suppes et al., 2001)

Formal, validated structured diagnostic interviews include the Structured Clinical Interview for DSM-IV-TR (SCID; First, Spitzer, Gibbon, & Williams, 2002) and the briefer Mini-International Neuropsychiatric Interview (MINI; Sheehan et al., 1998). Turning to these methods can be especially useful when the diagnostic picture is unclear or complicated by multiple medical and psychiatric comorbidities.

METHODS FOR MEASURING ILLNESS SEVERITY

In addition to the interview methods used to make the diagnosis of bipolar disorder, there are a number of both interview and self-report scales useful in assessing the *severity* of depression and mania/hypomania. These scales are not a substitute for a formal diagnostic procedure, but can be very helpful in monitoring treatment progress. Interview scales to assess the severity of depression include the Hamilton Depression Rating Scale in both its original 17-item (Hamilton, 1960) version and in any of the expanded versions that include the anergic symptoms that are frequently observed in bipolar depression, (e.g., Thase, Frank, Mallinger, Hamer, & Kupfer, 1992), as well as the Inventory of Depressive Symptoms (IDS; Rush et al., 1986). The IDS has the advantage of including both an interview and a self-report format. The two most often used interview scales to assess severity of mania are the Bech–Rafaelsen Mania Scale (Bech, Bolwig, Kramp, & Rafaelsen, 1979) and the Young Mania Rating Scale (YMRS; Young, Biggs, Ziegler, & Meyer, 1978). The Bech–Rafaelsen has the advantage of following the general format of the Hamilton and can be efficiently completed together with the Hamilton; however, the YMRS may be more appropriate for the assessment of mania/hypomania in the outpatient setting.

Self-report inventories for assessing severity of depression include the original Beck Depression Inventory (BDI; Beck, Ward, Mendelson, Mock, & Erbaugh, 1961) and its updated version, the BDI II (Beck, Steer, & Brown, 1996), as well as the longer (IDS) and shorter forms of the Inventory of Depressive Symptoms (QIDS; Rush et al., 2003). To our knowledge, no one has yet demonstrated the validity and reliability of a self-report scale to assess severity of mania/hypomania. Given the strong tendency of individuals to deny manic/hypomanic symptoms, the lack of insight that accompanies mania, and the psychotic nature of many manic episodes, this is not entirely surprising.

We have found that a helpful tool for obtaining a picture of the lifetime presence of both depressive and manic/hypomanic symptomatology is a self-report instrument that takes a spectrum approach to assessment of symptomatology. The MOODS-SR (Cassano et al., 1999a, 2002; Fagiolini et al., 1999) queries patients about the *lifetime* experience of a range of both typical and atypical mood symptoms and behavioral tendencies in both the depressive and manic domains and, in addition, inquires about the sensitivity of the individual to rhythm disturbances. The full series of Spectrum assessment instruments including the Panic Spectrum Assessment (PAS-SR–Cassano, et al., 1999b) referred to below, as well as information on their scoring, can be obtained from the Spectrum Project website at www.spectrum-project.org.

COMMON AXIS I COMORBIDITIES IN PATIENTS WITH BIPOLAR DISORDER

Bipolar disorder can present with a lifetime comorbidity of a variety of Axis I conditions, including anxiety disorders, eating disorders, and a host of other diagnoses. Probably the most common Axis I comorbidity seen in patients with bipolar disorder (and perhaps associated genetically with bipolar disorder) is panic disorder. In addition, many bipolar I patients who do not meet lifetime criteria for panic disorder will nonetheless report a lifetime history characterized by substantial evidence of panic and panic-like symptomatology, which we refer to as panic spectrum disorder (Cassano et al., 1997). Indeed, we found that in a group of bipolar I disorder patients whom we studied, although less than 15% met lifetime criteria for *panic disorder,* about one half reported a lifetime history of impairing *panic symptomatology* (Frank et al., 2002). Knowledge about the nature of your patient's panic comorbidity will be important inasmuch as it can have profound effects on medication adherence. Patients with lifetime panic disorder or panic spectrum comorbidity appear to be much more sensitive to and fearful of any perturbation in their somatic state, unusually sensitive to the side effects of medication, and thus require much more measured and careful upward titration of any psychoactive compound. You may find it useful to give your patient the self-report version of the assessment we have developed for the presence of lifetime panic spectrum (Cassano et al., 2002) in order to determine the extent to which he or she has experienced panic spectrum symptomatology.

Equally common among patients with bipolar disorder are *alcohol and substance abuse or dependence*. Many theories have been offered to explain this association. These include genetic association of the conditions, efforts on the part of the patient to self-medicate, and attempts to mimic the manic state, usually through the use of cocaine or amphetamines. Some bipolar patients who use drugs or alcohol when in acute episodes of mania or depression seem to be able to abstain when given appropriate treatment for their bipolar disorder. Others whose substance use is more lifelong will require specific treatment for this comorbidity.

For several reasons, our stand has always been that *any* alcohol or substance use is a bad idea for patients with bipolar disorder. All psychoactive substances have rebound effects on mood that make their use a temporary solution that is followed by a bigger problem. Patients who are taking medications other than lithium are already giving their liver extra work to do. It doesn't need more. Finally, alcohol and most illegal substances have negative effects on sleep architecture, robbing patients of the deep sleep that those with any mood disorder badly need.

Substantial numbers of patients with bipolar disorder also meet the criteria for *posttraumatic stress disorder* (PTSD), often directly as a result of their experience of bipolar disorder. Involuntary hospitalizations, common in this population, often constitute highly traumatic experiences that leave patients with all the criterion symptoms of PTSD. In addition, the poor judgment characteristic of mania often leads to involvement in situations that are dangerous and result in highly traumatic experiences. Finally, simply learning that one has a lifelong psychotic disorder can, in and of itself, constitute a trauma. Patients with bipolar disorder often report reexperiencing and other PTSD-like symptoms in association with learning of their bipolar I diagnosis.

It is also important to know about any present or past *eating disorders* your patient may have experienced. Any comorbid disorder that involves vomiting or extensive exercise can present special additional risks to patients taking lithium. Unlike other pharmacological treatments used in mood disorders, lithium is excreted by the kidneys, and fluid balance is essential to the maintenance of appropriate blood levels. Patients who vomit (either as a result of an eating disorder or as a result of a gastrointestinal infection) can become toxic in a matter of hours. The same is true of patients who become fluid deprived through extensive exercise or strenuous outdoor work in high temperatures. Preoccupation with body shape and weight not only has a strong association with negative mood states, which is relevant for the treatment of patients with bipolar disorder, but may seriously interfere with medication adherence either because the patient believes or actually sees that there is an association between the treatments prescribed and weight gain. Like panic symptomatology, eating disorder symptoms may also present in softer, subsyndromal forms (see Mauri et al., 2000) that can complicate the treatment of bipolar disorder. A self-report assessment of such anorexic–bulimic spectrum symptomatology (ABS-SR) is also available at www.spectrum-project.org.

As noted earlier, bipolar disorder in children can sometimes be mistaken for *attention-deficit/hyperactivity disorder* (*ADHD*); however, 40–80% of children and teens with bipolar disorder also have comorbid ADHD, and many adults with bipolar disorder are still struggling with the consequences of comorbid ADHD. Thus, your adolescent or adult patients may tell you that they also have or had ADHD. Evaluating the validity of this claim may be important in helping your IPSRT patient, especially if the focus of treatment is a role transition involving academic or work roles. Although you may not be an expert on ADHD, if you believe that the diagnosis is credible and the disorder is still active in your patient, you should make certain that he or she is also receiving appropriate treatment for ADHD. For successful treatment in children and adolescents with bipolar disorder and ADHD, both conditions need to be addressed with the best current treatments available. The diagnosis of ADHD in adults remains a somewhat controversial one, but it does appear to be gaining more acceptance. In some communities, clinicians are offering specific interventions for ADHD in adults.

AXIS II COMORBIDITIES

As implied in the preceding section on differential diagnosis, the question of Axis II comorbidity with bipolar disorder is a complex one. Most often patients with bipolar disorder who qualify for an Axis II diagnosis will qualify for one of the diagnoses in the Axis II Cluster B (borderline, antisocial, narcissistic, or dramatic personality disorder). Whether meeting *criteria* for one of these Axis II diagnoses represents a true comorbidity, or simply reflects the fact that there is a substantial amount of overlap between the symptoms required for a diagnosis of bipolar disorder and the symptoms required for any of these Axis II diagnoses, remains unclear at this point. For example, it is not difficult to see how the mood instability associated with bipolar disorder may be mistaken for the mood instability of borderline personality disorder. Yet there are patients who endorse essentially all of the symptoms of bipolar illness *and* all of the symptoms of borderline personality disorder, including those that do not overlap with bipolar disorder, such as the prototypic borderline self-injury. Again, knowing this about your patients can be quite important in how you support them in regard to their pharmacotherapy regimen. In our experience, those patients who actually suffer from *both* bipolar disorder and borderline personality disorder are not helped and are often made more symptomatic by many of the traditional pharmacotherapy regimens offered to patients with bipolar I disorder. Should a patient qualify for both of these diagnoses, in your role as the patient's coach and advocate in the pharmacotherapy realm, you may need to help your patient to obtain pharmacotherapy that actually makes him or her feel better and not worse. In our experience, the anticonvulsant lamotragine often has beneficial effects with such patients, whereas other more traditional mood stabilizers and antidepressants do not.

Patients with a long history of bipolar disorder with many manias can also present with what looks like avoidant personality disorder or even social phobia. Usually such presentations represent conditions that are secondary to patients' embarrassment about their past manic behavior and wariness about the potential for social involvement to cause new episodes of mania.

MEDICAL COMORBIDITIES

For reasons that are not entirely clear—perhaps it is a matter of genetic association, perhaps a matter of the wear and tear caused by the illness itself, perhaps a matter of the long-term effects of some of the treatments for the illness—patients with bipolar disorder tend to suffer from many more medical conditions than either their counterparts with unipolar disorder or nonpsychiatrically ill persons in the general community. Of particular note is the frequency with which thyroid disease, diabetes, cardiovascular disease, hypertension, obesity, and skin conditions like eczema and psoriasis are observed in patients with bipolar disorder, particularly bipolar I disorder. This makes it particularly important that the patient is receiving good medical care on a regular basis. Part of your responsibility as an advocate for your bipolar patients is to be certain that they obtain such care and that they follow up on the recommendations of their medical doctor. It also means being aware of the medications your patients are taking for any such condition and the possible interactions that could occur with the medications being prescribed for their bipolar disorder. Even if you are not a physician yourself, providing adequate care, particularly to patients with bipolar I disorder, means being well informed about all the medications your patients are taking and their possible effects on your patients' physical and psychological well-being.

FINAL THOUGHTS

The initial and ongoing assessment of the patient with bipolar disorder is a complex process. If your work to date has been primarily with the outpatient treatment of nonpsychotic mood and anxiety disorders, taking on patients with bipolar disorder may require the acquisition of additional diagnostic skills and additional knowledge about the pharmacotherapy of bipolar disorder and a host of possible comorbid psychiatric and physical conditions. With respect to diagnosis, there is no substitute for experience. The more patients you see with bipolar disorders, the sharper your diagnostic skills and intuition will become. The patients themselves are often great teachers, especially those who have suffered with the disorder for many years. Listen to their stories and you will learn a great deal. As to information about specific medications, medication interactions, and medical conditions, today high-quality information is available in each of these areas through the Web. Information for clinicians about a range of medical conditions, as well as about medications and drug interactions, can be obtained at www.medicinenet.com, www.medscape.com, and my.webmd.com. An excellent source of new information about bipolar disorder (and one that you may want to share with your patients) is McMan's *Depression and Bipolar Weekly* available at www. mcmanweb.com.

SIX

The Individualized Case Formulation
History Taking and the Interpersonal Inventory

When psychodynamically trained psychotherapists talk about a case formulation, they are usually referring to a *theoretical* formulation that helps them to understand how a given patient came to think, feel, and act in particular ways. In IPT and IPSRT, a case formulation refers to something quite different. An IPSRT case formulation is a *practical* working map of what is going on in the patient's life and what you and he or she intend to do to change the unpleasant or symptom-producing aspects of the patient's life. The key tools in arriving at an IPSRT case formulation are the history taking, the interpersonal inventory, and the preintervention completion of the Social Rhythm Metric. This chapter focuses on the use of each of these tools.

Even at the most basic level, with the most straightforward of cases, IPSRT implies through its focus on five different interpersonal problem areas (grief, role transitions, role disputes, interpersonal deficits, and grief for the lost healthy self) that cases must be formulated on the basis of the particular problems that are related to the individual patient's mania or depression. Individualized case formulation is also critical because patients with bipolar disorder present for treatment with a great diversity of past histories and current problems, as well as with vastly different levels of knowledge and insight about their condition. At the end of this process you should be able to articulate a case formulation that states in general what the relationship has been among what kinds of interpersonal problems, what kinds of external demands, what kinds of rhythm disruptions, and what kinds of symptoms throughout this particular patient's history of bipolar illness. Even more important, you should be able to state specifically what interpersonal or social role problems are contributing to what social rhythm disruptions leading to what kinds of symptoms currently. You should then be able to articulate what your plan will be (with your patient's consent) for addressing the interpersonal problems and for modifying his or her social rhythms, with what expected result in his or her current symptoms. Given your patient's particular history, you should also have an idea of what the two of you will need to look out for in both the interpersonal and social rhythm realms in order to protect your patient from future episodes of illness. When IPSRT does not go well, it is often because the case formulation is not correct and the problem area selected is not the right one. Thus, case formulation is a critical first step in the conduct of IPSRT.

As mentioned earlier, IPSRT is a four-phase treatment. The entire first phase is, in a sense, devoted to the process of case formulation. As you proceed through the subsequent phases of treatment, and as your patient's clinical state changes, you may find that you need to adjust your formulation or, sometimes, reconceptualize the case entirely.

In the initial phase you will focus on taking the history of your patient's illness, educating your patient about bipolar disorder, completing what is known as the "interpersonal inventory," and identifying the interpersonal problem area or areas that will become the focus of your interpersonal interventions. It is these initial activities that allow you to arrive at an initial case formulation. Irrespective of whether IPSRT is begun while your patient is acutely ill or initiated as a maintenance treatment during a euthymic period, the patient's introduction to IPSRT and the process of case formulation generally occur over the course of three to four consecutive weekly sessions. In some complex cases or with patients who are very depressed and uncommunicative, you may find that you need more than four sessions, but rarely will you be able to accomplish these initial goals in fewer than three sessions.

If this is your patient's first treatment for his or her bipolar disorder, you may need to spend a considerable amount of time teaching him or her about the nature of the illness and helping your patient to accept what is clearly a very frightening diagnosis. This was certainly the case with Tad, the young artist whom you read about in Chapter 1. When he entered IPSRT treatment, he had never heard of bipolar disorder and had no context whatever for understanding what was happening to him. Thus, one aspect of the individualized case formulation for Tad was that he was lacking information about mood disorders and that his treatment plan would thus need to include extensive education about mood disorders, starting at the most basic level.

Other patients begin IPSRT having been in treatment for many years and knowing a great deal about the illness. In such cases, the psychoeducation may require less time or may begin at a much more sophisticated level than it could with Tad. Nonetheless, it is important for you to understand each patient's conceptualization of the illness. Those patients who received their diagnoses many years ago may have done a substantial amount of reading and talking with others about bipolar disorder. Such individuals often have a large body of correct information and a deep understanding of the illness and how it has affected their lives. However, some patients have acquired numerous misconceptions about their illness and its treatment. It then becomes your obligation to begin work on correcting these misconceptions in the early phase of the treatment. Still others, like Jill whom you also read about in the first chapter, may have largely avoided the topic. Despite having had bipolar disorder for many years and despite being otherwise well read and well informed, patients like Jill may be relatively naive about the illness and may require extensive education about their illness.

TAKING THE HISTORY OF THE ILLNESS

As mentioned earlier, whenever possible, IPSRT begins with a review of the patient's experience of the illness. This review covers symptomatic, social rhythm disruption, and interpersonal aspects of earlier episodes, with particular emphasis on the most recent episodes. The philosophy of and rationale for IPSRT, which grow out of the social *zeitgeber* hypothesis (Ehlers, Frank, et al., 1988) described in Chapter 2, assume a close and interdependent relationship between interpersonal distress and disruption in the social rhythms of the patient's life. In taking the history, therefore, you will want to look for any evidence of alterations or disruptions in your patient's routine of daily life and interpersonal interactions that *preceded* the development of symptoms. With your patient's permission, you may choose to involve a family member or close friend in this process, especially if the patient has limited recall of his or her ascent into mania. Depending on the nature of that individual's relationship with your patient, this can either be done in a conjoint session or in a separate interview, as long as there is clear agreement between you and your patient, as well as between the patient and family member or friend as to the parameters with respect to confidentiality.

When the illness history cannot be taken at the outset of treatment because the patient is in crisis or is too ill to be able to provide the information, it is best to try to gather the history as soon as possible. It may be possible to piece together some aspects of the history from your patient's records, if these are obtainable, and then feed this information back to the patient as you begin to develop the rationale for the changes you are asking the patient to make. Or you may be able to obtain considerable information from family members. If the patient is your only resource, as soon as it seems reasonable, you will want to turn to the history taking because it generally proves to be your best ammunition in making the case for the treatment. If doing the history taking all at once seems likely to prove too stressful or difficult for the patient, you can plan on breaking it up into smaller chunks, devoting 15 minutes or so at the beginning or end of several sessions to obtaining the information you need.

The treatment session or sessions focusing on illness history and the interpersonal inventory are of primary importance in helping you and your patient to understand the extent to which rhythm disruption has been associated with episode onsets and which aspects of the patient's interpersonal relationships may have contributed to the onset and/or exacerbation of the current episode.

As mentioned in Chapter 4, teasing apart the relationship between early symptoms and any lifestyle alterations that may have preceded those symptoms is often difficult. For example, decreased sleep is both *a core symptom of* and *a trigger for* mania or hypomania (Wehr, Sack, & Rosenthal, 1987). The role of increased sleep and inactivity in precipitating depression is less clear; but it does seem to be the case that when activity is increased, mood improvement frequently ensues (Beck et al., 1979). Although there is no direct evidence that *oversleeping* leads to depressive symptoms, numerous studies have demonstrated the strong, although transient, antidepressant effect of *sleep deprivation* (Gillin, Buchsbaum, Wu, Clark, & Bunney, 2001; Wirz-Justice & Van den Hoofdakker, 1999).

When carefully taken histories are examined, it is often possible to separate externally caused disruptions in routine from prodromal symptoms of mania or depression. In taking the history, you should therefore concentrate on whether your patient, for example, noted a gradual decrease in sleep over the course of several days or weeks. Or, was it the case that the patient experienced an externally driven *need* to stay up most or all of the night (in order to write a paper or speech, prepare for an examination, or as a result of long distance or transoceanic travel) just prior to the onset of a manic episode? In the first case, the decrease in sleep was likely an early *symptom* of a developing mania. In the second case, the loss of sleep was likely a *cause* of the subsequent mania, a cause that you and your patient can work to avoid in the future. In the history-taking process, you will also want to probe for the earliest observable symptoms of the most recent episode, which may have nothing to do with sleep, and for what your patient perceives as the characteristic early signs of past manias or depressions, attempting to get a clear picture of how each kind of episode typically begins for the patient. For some patients mania begins with a little uncharacteristic suspiciousness or paranoia. For others, it may be that colors seem brighter and smells seem stronger. Early signs of depression for one patient may differ dramatically from those for another, but generally each patient has his or her own characteristic pattern.

If you think back to the two cases described in Chapter 1, you can see how even at the history-taking stage you would begin to formulate these two cases differently. Jill's episode onsets seem very clearly linked to hormonal events that had routine-disrupting aspects to them and, to a lesser extent, to external events that disrupted her routine apart from any reproductive events of her own. She also seemed to have some seasonal pattern to her mood disorder, at least earlier in her life. Tad's episodes, in contrast, seem clearly linked to unstable social rhythms and social and intellectual overstimulation. Information obtained from the history taking suggests different emphases for these two different cases.

THE ILLNESS HISTORY TIMELINE

In taking the history of a patient's illness, it is very helpful to construct a written timeline that includes episodes of illness, treatment, important life events, lifestyle alterations, and any other information you and your patient deem relevant to understanding the precipitants of episodes and the kinds of treatments have been helpful in the past. We see this as a key tool in the individual case formulation in IPSRT as well as a key tool in developing the rationale for the lifestyle changes you will be asking your patient to make. An example of such a timeline for Jill, the patient described at the beginning of Chapter 1, is provided in Figure 6.1.

The timeline we constructed begins with Jill's experiences of mild depression during high school, which seemed to have no particular social precipitants but did appear to be seasonal in occurrence. It then moves on to note the psychotic mixed state that followed the birth of her first child and notes her treatment with lithium and atypical neuroleptic at that time. It also records her employment status at the time of this episode. The timeline shows her complete recovery from the episode and then the depression that began with her visit to Seattle to help care for her brother and sister-in-law's child and all the disruptions in her routines that accompanied that visit. It also indicates how long it took for her to recover from that depression in the absence of any treatment and how the result of this episode caused her to move from her position as a university professor to the role of high school teacher. The timeline shows the mania associated with the birth of her second child and her second good response to the combination of lithium and atypical neuroleptic. It illustrates her period of stability following her commitment to consistent treatment with lithium and her continued employment during that period. It then denotes the mania associated with her miscarriage and the subsequent difficulties in bringing this mania under

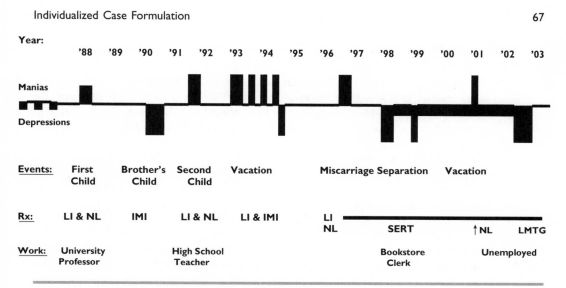

FIGURE 6.1. Example of an illness history timeline.

control prior to her treatment with electroconvulsive therapy. It also denotes the fact that following this episode, Jill did not return to the euthymia that had characterized much of her interepisode functioning up to this point, the further decline in her employment status, and the deterioration of her marriage, associated with the fact that she never fully returned to the euthymic state that had characterized her interepisode functioning up to that point.

A timeline like this can be very useful not only for educating the patient about his or her disorder, but also for developing the rationale for the social rhythm aspects of IPSRT with the patient. Each of Jill's manias seemed to have been precipitated by the overwhelming hormonal changes (and sleep deprivation) associated with reproductive events. Her depressions, in contrast, appear to have been associated with periods of relative inactivity that were characterized by a lack of structure and routine. Even her marital separation, which undoubtedly was characterized by much sadness as well as routine disruption, was associated with major changes in the structure of her day-to-day routines.

EDUCATING YOUR PATIENT ABOUT BIPOLAR DISORDER

During both the history taking and the timeline construction and, in fact, throughout the initial phase of treatment, you will be ascertaining how much your patient knows about the disorder and how much he or she understands about how interpersonal problems and lifestyle disruption may have been related to the onset and continuation of episodes. Even patients who have suffered from bipolar disorder for many years and who have read extensively about the disorder may not see these connections. These early sessions offer an opportunity to help your patient to see the links between interpersonal problems, rhythm disruption, and symptom exacerbation. Thus, even while you are still formulating the case and your treatment plan, you can begin to weave some psychoeducation into the treatment process.

CASE EXAMPLE

Alison is a 38-year-old divorced female who entered IPSRT treatment following her fourth manic episode. In Session 2, she and her therapist were reviewing the events that had led up to each of her manic episodes. Although she had never made the connection previously, it became apparent that the common factor preceding each of her episodes was sleep deprivation, often combined with missing a single dose of lithium. At her job as a graphic designer, Alison was often required to work late hours in order to complete projects. On the nights prior to three of her onsets of mania, her boss insisted that she stay up all night in order to meet a deadline. On each of these occasions, she also neglected to take her evening dose of lithium. Her fourth episode followed a night when she had been kept up all night by persistent nausea and vomiting related to an intestinal flu. Although she had taken her lithium dose prior to the onset of the vomiting, probably little of it remained in her system. The similarity of the events leading up to each of her episodes was obvious when she reviewed them, but because she had been working in different settings for different individuals at the times of onset, she failed to see the connection between her sleep deprivation and the onset of her manic episodes.

Although it may be painful and difficult for the patient, in taking the history it is important that you explore all aspects of both depressive and manic or hypomanic episodes, as this will help in building the rationale for the changes that you will ask your patient to make in his or her lifestyle. It is also very important to make explicit the evidence of dysfunction, socially inappropriate behavior, or other behaviors that have caused your patient embarrassment or sadness, financial loss, or loss of professional or social standing. Many patients with bipolar disorder will almost proudly regale you with tales of the outrageous things they did during their worst episodes, but this may be difficult information to obtain, especially if your patient is depressed or is not yet entirely comfortable with you. If you suspect that there may have been such negative consequences to episodes, you should try, in the gentlest and most supportive way possible, to explore what the impact of episodes might have been on how he or she got along at work; for example, did the mania or the depression lead to any conflicts with coworkers or superiors? You might also explore whether this was a particularly difficult time in terms of family relationships, what the patient thinks the impact of the episode might have been on close family members or friends, whether there was anything that the patient did during the episode that he or she now regrets, or whether he or she failed to do something that should have been done. In taking the histories of patients with many prior episodes, it is often possible to chart gradual, but significant downward social mobility and increasing underemployment over time, as was the case with Jill. Thus, particularly with patients who have been ill for many years, you may wish to include employment and other indices of socioeconomic status, such as place of residence, on the timeline.

After such changes are identified, many patients spontaneously comment on the tremendous personal costs of the disorder. If your patient seems unable to grasp the full impact of the disorder on his or her life, you can query the patient directly, asking the patient to describe how his or her professional or occupational standing might differ today if he or she had never had an affective episode. What sort of work does she imagine she would be doing? What kind of compensation does he think he would be getting? What sort of lifestyle does she believe she would be leading?

You need to be prepared for the emotional impact that recognizing the full cost of the disorder may have on patients and should gauge carefully your patient's readiness to hear and to assimilate this information. If your patient seems particularly distressed, you may want to plan a phone contact between this visit and the subsequent one.

With younger patients and those with few episodes, a slightly altered process may be possible in which you and the patient jointly develop an extended scenario about future occupational attainment, as it might be anticipated both with and without subsequent episodes of illness.

CASE EXAMPLE

Andy is a 28-year-old single male with a 13-year history of bipolar I disorder. His bipolar illness has a seasonal pattern. The depressive episodes have occurred almost every fall and remitted in early spring. Each summer since high school he has experienced at least a moderate level of hypomania, clearly noticeable to friends and family. Both of his fully manic episodes have occurred in summer, and, fortunately, neither has had a seriously damaging effect on his personal or academic life. Rather, he and his IPSRT therapist spent much of the first few sessions discussing the impact of his seasonal depressions on his life, especially on his academic career. In high school, though he did poorly during the first term, he always managed to bring his grades up by the end of the school year. His uneven record meant he did not get into the kind of college that his intelligence and SAT scores would have warranted, but he did enroll at a local junior college after high school. Throughout his late teens and early 20s, Andy enrolled in college several different times. Things would start off well enough, but by the middle of the fall semester he would become immobilized by his anergia, find it impossible to concentrate, stop showing up for class, and, eventually, he would then drop out of school. His well-meaning but frustrated patents accused him variously of being lazy, of being unable to finish anything he started, and of just wanting to be in college to "party on their dollar." In fact, though, he has always been willing to work to try to support himself, even if it was at a menial job well below his level of intellectual competence, when he was well. He has held a variety of service and clerical jobs over the years, all singularly unfulfilling. For the past 4 years, however, he has been very active in volunteering for a nonprofit organization that organizes tutoring for elementary school kids who are having academic difficulties, but whose parents are unable to give them help. He enjoys this work immensely. Indeed, it is the first thing in his life that he has ever been truly and persistently enthusiastic about. Were it not for his bipolar illness, his career goal would be to finish college and become an elementary school teacher; however, he is currently convinced that that his bipolar illness will probably prevent him from reaching this goal. In discussing the limitations his illness has placed on his academic and career pursuits, Andy is aware that, without a major change in the course of his illness, it is unlikely he will be able to finish school or even to lead the organization he volunteers for—another of his dreams.

At this point it is your job to help your patient make a realistic assessment of what can and what cannot change. Andy is likely to remain vulnerable to fall depressions and spring/summer hypomanias for the rest of his life. However, you can legitimately offer the possibility that with appropriate pharmacotherapy and appropriate self-discipline on Andy's part, he may be able to make up for some of the lost time he has experienced and, ultimately, not only realize his goal of having a leadership position in his volunteer organization but also complete his higher education and substantially alter the trajectory that his life is currently on.

As Andy's IPSRT therapist, your job would be to assess whether it might be possible for Andy to achieve his goals with the right medication regimen and a very gradual reentry into college work. This assessment may actually take many months to complete, perhaps including a trial run by taking a single course at school. If this process indicates that finishing college is simply not possible for a patient like Andy, then your job is to help him establish a series of realistic goals, given the limits imposed by his illness. If, however, you find that with appropriate medication, attention to the regularity of his routines, and a good deal of support from you and his family, it seems as though eventually completing college might be a possibility, you would then map out a program for very gradually achieving that goal. (Family members can be engaged as "ancillary members" of the treatment team, which may include the psychiatrist or group of psychiatrists who are responsible for pharmacotherapy and any other medical or other specialists involved in the patient's care or social and occupational rehabilitation or monitoring.) Depending on how things progress, it might be a program in which study always remains a part-time process and is coupled with a part-time job that helps to anchor Andy's self-scheduling. If he does extremely well with part-time study and seems able to discipline himself with respect to his routines, it might eventually mean full-time studies. The point is that, in contrast to how you are likely to proceed in the short-term therapies for most mood and anxiety disorders, in IPSRT the time frame is greatly extended and you are constantly assessing and reassessing how each patient is responding to your interventions and what those assessments tell you about long-term goals.

During the history taking, a similar process can be followed with respect to understanding the relationship between your patient's mood and the nature of his or her personal relationships once you have completed an interpersonal inventory (see the discussion in the next section). You will want to ask the older patient to speculate about what family relationships and friendships might be like today had he or she never suffered from bipolar illness. A younger patient can be asked to imagine the impact of many subsequent episodes on the relationships he or she currently values.

In helping your patient to see the costs incurred as a result of his or her bipolar illness, you are building the case for the difficult changes you are asking that patient to make. In doing so, however, you are walking a fine line between helping the patient to see the need for change and making the patient feel so discouraged that he or she is not motivated to change. Knowing exactly where you should be on this fine line is further complicated by the mood instability that characterizes the disorder itself. If the patient is euthymic or only mildly hypomanic when you are making your case for change, you can be much more forceful and assertive about the difficulties and costs associated with the illness. If, however, the patient is somewhat depressed at the time you are making the case for the treatment, you must be much more careful in order to avoid further demoralizing an already demoralized individual.

CASE EXAMPLE

Steve is a 50-year-old single white male with a 12-year history of bipolar disorder. Steve was a high-ranking civil servant working in local government in another part of the country, but for the past year he has been unemployed. Steve has suffered four manic episodes over the past 12 years. His manias have severely impaired his interpersonal relationships. During his manic episodes he becomes intolerably intrusive when interacting with people. At these times, his interpersonal relationships are characterized by irritability and argumentative behavior. He becomes involved in excessive planning and participates in an endless stream of career-related and social activities. He reports frequent attempts to recontact old friends and former coworkers, calling them at odd hours. His friends have commented to him on the inappropriateness of his behavior, his loud and rapid speech, and their difficulty in following his monologues. His manic behavior has caused significant problems with his former coworkers and bosses. As a result (during his fourth episode of mania), he was terminated from his position. Because this termination did occur while he was in a manic state, he became consumed with trying to get his position back. He was aggressive, hostile, intrusive, and obnoxiously demanding. He contacted influential people who were only casual acquaintances. These people were surprised and angry at his odd behavior and perseverance. For the most part, they have severed all ties with him. In retrospect, he recognizes that his judgment was very poor and that he behaved in ways he now regrets.

As he looks back on his behavior during these manias, Steve acknowledges how detrimental they have been to him. His bipolar illness has created severe problems with regard to his interpersonal relationships and his career. He recognizes that if his mood had been stable throughout this period, he would still have his friends and social support network, as well as the job that he greatly enjoyed. He now sees that his bipolar disorder has caused him much embarrassment and pain in regard to his ability to maintain relationships and behave appropriately with his coworkers and friends. As a 50-year-old man, he is ashamed that his mother and sister are now his only real social supports. He believes that if he did not suffer from bipolar illness, his social supports would consist of the large network of friends and colleagues he once had. He might also have been able to maintain a long-term relationship with a woman who would have provided him with additional emotional support and security.

If Steve were your patient, your task would be to assess whether the damage he has done is truly irreparable, or whether it might be possible—gradually—to reconnect with some of his former support network and, perhaps, even to return to his former job or something like it. This will require gathering a lot of information about the specific disputes that occurred during his mania, whether his former friends and colleagues completely fail to understand what was happening during Steve's manias and are truly unwilling to have any contact with him or whether, as is often the case, he is simply too embarrassed by his behavior to want to contact them or too afraid of the potential rejection to try. What may complicate this process for you is that frequently patients have only a partial recollection of what happened during severe episodes of mania and that even what they can remember is often filtered through the very poor judgment characteristic of mania. Still, with patience, it is usually possible to help your patient make a realistic assessment of which, if any, relationships are forever damaged and which have good potential for repair.

TAKING THE INTERPERSONAL INVENTORY

Of all the aspects of the initial phase of IPSRT, it is the interpersonal inventory that is most critical to the individual case formulation. The term "interpersonal inventory" simply refers to a review of the important relationships in a patient's life, past and present (Klerman et al., 1984). This inventory focuses on understanding what the nature of these relationships has been, whether there are any consistent positive or negative patterns in the patient's relationships, and, particularly, whether problems in any of these relationships are linked to the onset or persistence of the most recent episode of illness, either through their psychological impact or through their impact on social rhythms. The completion of the interpersonal inventory is the last part of the extended history-taking process and leads directly to the individual case formulation in IPSRT.

Because the emphasis in interpersonal psychotherapy is clearly on the very recent past, the present, and the near future, you begin the interpersonal inventory with the important relationships in the patient's life at the time that the patient enters treatment. So, for example, in completing an interpersonal inventory for Jill (Chapter 1), you would start with a detailed exploration of Jill's relationship with her estranged husband. You would want to know how frequently they have contact, what the nature of those contacts is, and how they relate to one another with respect to parenting their children. You would inquire about the frequency of arguments and, most important, about the nature of Jill's feelings for her husband at the present time. You would also explore Jill's perception of her husband's feelings for her, trying to determine whether the relationship really is completely dissolved or whether, in fact, despite their 3-year separation, they are at somewhat of an impasse with respect to the dissolution of their marriage. You would then go on to explore the development of that important relationship, how Jill and her husband met, what their dating experience was like, and what the nature of their relationship was in the early years of their marriage. Although Jill's children are still quite young, you would want to know about the nature of her relationship with each of her boys and get a clear sense of how the boys are currently functioning. Given Jill's markedly deteriorated state, you might well include her husband in part of this assessment in order to explore what, if any, interest he might have in a marital reconciliation and how he views his role with respect to Jill, her illness, and their children.

Moving on from these key relationships, you would explore the nature of Jill's relationship with each of her parents, going back as far as seems necessary to understand the full nature of each of these relationships. Knowing that Jill had once been close to her brother and her brother's wife, this would be another relationship that you would explore in depth, with the hope that they might become an important source of support despite how far away they are. Finally, you would try to explore the nature of Jill's relationships with friends and coworkers, both present and past, to determine something about her capacities for forming and sustaining relationships prior to the development of her illness and how the illness has affected those capacities.

In Jill's case, such an exploration would reveal that a very strong and reciprocal affective bond existed between Jill and her husband. Each cared deeply about the other but was completely bewildered as to how to relate to one another in the face of her bipolar illness. The interpersonal inventory would also reveal her real feelings of inadequacy as a mother at this point in time and the extent to which her mood disorder had completely undermined her sense of competence as a parent. The inventory would also reveal her somewhat more superficial relationship with each of her parents. Although her mother and father could be counted on for instrumental support (her mother with the care of the children and her father with her financial concerns, transportation needs, etc.), neither of her parents had a real capacity for emotional support. In contrast, Jill and her sister-in-law had been able to maintain a confiding relationship in spite of her illness, and her sister-in-law remains someone whom she can count on for unconditional affection, empathy, and understanding. The only problem was that her sister-in-law was thousands of miles away. The interpersonal inventory would also reveal that as a younger woman, Jill had many close friends and several with whom she had a truly confiding relationship. But, unlike her relationship with her sister-in-law who had stuck by her through the worst of her depressions, Jill's friends had more or less fallen by the wayside as Jill failed to reciprocate their offers of friendship. Whether any of these friendships could be resurrected once Jill was feeling better had been a question in the therapist's mind; however, by the time the interpersonal inventory was completed, the therapist had a picture of someone who clearly had the capacity for satisfying interpersonal relationships when depression was not depriving her of all emotional energy and making her so prickly and irritable that she actually found it easier to be alone.

Tad presents a different kind of challenge in taking the interpersonal inventory. Although chronologically 18 years of age at the time he entered treatment, developmentally Tad was more like a 15-year-old. Further complicating the situation was the fact that all of his important relationships were back home in Alabama, but his current interpersonal context was the city where he was attending college and being treated. The interpersonal inventory needed to begin with an exploration of his relationship with each of his parents and revealed a strongly supportive relationship with his mother, of whom he was extremely fond. His relationship with his stern, disciplinarian father was not nearly as good. Tad had always been a disappointment to his father, who devalued Tad's artistic accomplishments much as he yearned for a son more interested in "masculine" pursuits. His mother, in contrast, remained close and very supportive of him and worked constantly to try to improve the relationship between father and son. Although Tad had been at college for only a matter of months when he entered treatment, he had, in fact, formed many strong, supportive relationships since entering school. Not surprisingly, his fellow art students were much more understanding of his bizarre behavior than his postal worker father had been. Because he never became irritable or angry in his manias, Tad had not really alienated any of these friends, each of whom was anxious to know what they could do to help Tad out of his postmania depression and facilitate his reentry into college life. Several of these friends accompanied Tad to his clinic appointments and represented an important resource in the conduct of his treatment. Tad's romantic relationships, like those of many young men, proved a much more difficult challenge for the therapist and for Tad's mood. The interpersonal inven-

tory revealed that Tad had always been attracted to very flamboyant and not particularly caring or supportive partners. Their frequent rejections and his dramatic reconcili-
ations with them did little to add to Tad's mood stability. The therapist identified this as
an area that would require considerable work in the future, once his role transition to
being a stable college student had been completed.

There is no set formula for taking an interpersonal inventory. The most skillful
IPSRT therapists do it in an apparently conversational manner; however, they are
working from a kind of implicit interview outline that begins with current close relationships and moves on to current more peripheral relationships and, finally, to important past relationships. To facilitate the training of new IPSRT therapists and to study
cross-cultural differences in the interpersonal problems of patients with bipolar disorder, we developed an interview guide for the interpersonal inventory (Andrade et al.,
2004). A copy of this interview guide is included in Appendix 5. Patients who have had
a good deal of experience in therapy will often more or less structure this part of the assessment for you. Patients with less treatment experience will need to be prompted by
direct questions, like those in the interview guide, so that by the time the interpersonal
inventory is completed, you have a clear picture of the people who are currently important to the patient, those who have been important to the patient in the past, and the nature of each of these relationships. In working with patients with bipolar disorder, it is
also important to inquire about important relationships that have ended or have been
abruptly cut off. Bipolar symptomatology often leads to such cutoffs either because the
other person has been so frightened by the nature of the patient's behavior, or because
the patient in an irritable, manic, or depressed state has ended all contact with the other
person. Thus, a final question at the conclusion of the interpersonal inventory might be,
"Is there anyone who was once quite important to you whom you no longer see or with
whom you no longer speak?" If a patient describes such a relationship, you will want
to explore whether reconnecting with this person might be beneficial to the patient.

As the preceding examples illustrate, it is important that you not only understand
the nature of a patient's current and past relationships, but also how relatives and
friends respond to the patient when he or she is symptomatic and what impact the illness has had on interpersonal relationships. Has it led to temporary disruptions or cutoffs? Has the patient become enmeshed with overinvolved, overresponsible family
members? Do relatives, friends, neighbors, or coworkers know about the patient's illness? How much do they know about the illness? How have they responded when the
patient has been ill? Do they respond differently when the patient is manic versus depressed, in terms of their willingness to provide support? Do they respond differently
to the patient when he or she is asymptomatic?

Although IPSRT distinguishes a small series of problem areas on which the treatment should be focused (grief, grief for the lost healthy self, role transitions, role disputes, and interpersonal deficits), the variety of issues that might be addressed within
these problem areas are as numerous as the patient population is complex. Often you
will see several problems that you think would be useful to address. Rather than trying
to work on multiple problems at the same time, however, we have generally tried to focus on one. We usually choose to begin with the problem most linked to the patient's
current symptoms or with the one most likely to facilitate engaging the patient in treatment. For example, at the point that Jill entered treatment, her case might be thought of
as one of interpersonal deficits. However, this is often a difficult place to *begin* treat-

ment and, unlike many people with interpersonal deficits, Jill has demonstrated the capacity for meaningful and supportive friendships in the past.

Probably a better place to engage a patient like Jill is with a focus on grief for the lost healthy self. Once Jill has been helped to mourn for her multiple lost opportunities and frustrated goals (and in Jill's case this could take a fair amount of time), the therapist is then faced with the challenge of deciding where to focus next. Is there enough of a relationship remaining with Jill's husband to conceptualize her case as a role dispute that has been in a 3-year phase of dissolution, but is not fully resolved? Would conceptualizing her case as a role transition from married to single life be more likely of benefit? Key to this decision would be a session or two with Jill's husband in which the therapist could assess his views on whether the marriage could ever be salvaged or whether the best that could be hoped for is a respectful relationship that would allow them to jointly parent their boys.

In taking the interpersonal inventory, many of us have found it useful to complete a genogram (a graph of all the patient's recent ancestors and descendents) before starting the inventory. This will ensure that no family members are missed in the inventory process. In the context of complex sets of relationships, such as occur when parents have been divorced and remarried or the patient has been in foster care, a genogram can help you to follow a complicated history and provide a quick reference guide to your patient's relationships as you proceed through treatment. An example of such a genogram is presented in Figure 6.2. Keep in mind that among some ethnic groups, such as African Americans and Hispanics, relationships with grandparents, aunts, and uncles may be more like those with parents and relationships with cousins may be

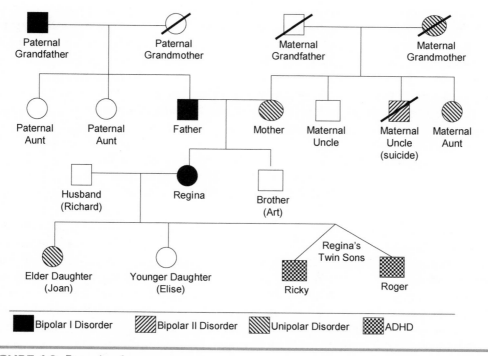

FIGURE 6.2. Example of a genogram.

more like those with siblings. Thus, understanding the nature of your patient's relationship to these individuals may be very important to effective treatment.

Once you have completed the interpersonal inventory, you should have most of the information you need to begin the process of case formulation and to present and discuss your initial formulation with your patient. In some cases, like Jill's for example, it may be necessary to include other people in one or two sessions before the case conceptualization can be considered complete.

In conceptualizing IPSRT cases, it is essential that you keep in mind that bipolar disorder is a lifelong and constantly evolving condition. Therefore, throughout IPSRT you will find that you are continually formulating and reformulating your conceptualization of your patient's needs and capacities and what the nature of your interventions should be.

IDENTIFICATION OF A PROBLEM AREA

After the interpersonal inventory is completed, you will want to determine which interpersonal issues are most central to your patient's current mood symptomatology. Again, this may be a problem that is either a likely *cause* of the current mood episode (e.g., a difficult role transition leading to an episode of mania) or an *effect* of the current episode (e.g., extreme overspending, leading to a marital role dispute and threatened separation). In either case, resolution of the interpersonal problem appears likely to lead to improvement in your patient's mood and functioning.

Under ideal circumstances, you and your patient will collaboratively identify a primary (and sometimes a secondary) problem area among the four interpersonal problems areas originally associated with interpersonal psychotherapy for unipolar disorder—unresolved grief, interpersonal disputes, role transition, and interpersonal deficits (cf. Klerman et al., 1984). For a full discussion of the conceptual basis for the interpersonal problem areas, see *Interpersonal Psychotherapy of Depression* (Klerman et al., 1984) and the *Comprehensive Guide to Interpersonal Psychotherapy* (Weissman et al., 2000). Extended descriptions of each of the interpersonal problem areas as they manifest themselves in patients with bipolar disorder are included in Chapter 9.

INITIATING THE SOCIAL RHYTHM METRIC
AND IDENTIFICATION OF GOALS
FOR RHYTHM STABILIZATION

The second major part of IPSRT case conceptualization has to do with the nature of the patient's social rhythms and the interventions that will be necessary to achieve social rhythm stability. As argued in Chapter 2, if loss of social *zeitgebers* and the presence of significant *zeitstörers* are important variables in triggering affective episodes in vulnerable individuals, then principles of social rhythm stabilization form an important part of treatment, particularly prophylactic treatment, and the nature of the patient's social routines forms an important part of your case concepualization. In order to evaluate the stability of social rhythms, we developed an instrument specifically designed to measure the rhythmicity of a person's daily life. This instrument, called the Social Rhythm Metric (SRM), tracks the timing of the occurrence of 15 prespecified activities and 2 individually selected activities (such as a particular leisure activity, prayer, or dog walking) that the person completing the instrument reports taking part in more days than not (Monk et al., 1990, 1991). The original version of the Social Rhythm Metric has been used in several different studies involving healthy controls (Monk et al., 1990), recovered depressed patients (Monk et al., 1991), depressed inpatients (Szuba, Yager, Guze, Allen, & Baxter, 1992), and healthy older people (Monk et al., 1992). On all forms of the SRM, a high score indicates a high degree of regularity in the timing of daily events, whereas a low score indicates irregularity or the absence of routine. Depressed inpatients were found to have a lower SRM score than healthy midlife community controls, and the older people (70+ years) had a higher than average SRM score.

We subsequently developed two new versions of the SRM, both for use in the treatment of individuals with bipolar disorder. The first of these adaptations, the SRM-II-17, was used in our initial study of IPSRT (see Appendix 3). We have demonstrated that the participation in IPSRT is associated with increases in the regularity of the activities recorded on the SRM-II. Then, because the 17-item version of the SRM-II proves impractical in many treatment contexts and because we found that most of the variance in the SRM score was accounted for by a small subset of the original 17 items (Monk et al., 2002), we developed a five-item version of the SRM-II (SRM-II-5; see Appendix 1), which inquires only about when the individual (1) got out of bed, (2) first had contact with another person, (3) started work, school, or housework, (4) had dinner, and (5) went to bed. This version is currently being used in the large national multicenter Systematic Treatment Enhancement Program (STEP-BD) study of treatments for bipolar disorder.

Many clinicians have found it useful to individualize the SRM to meet specific needs of particular patients. For example, for women who tend to have premenstrual exacerbation of mood (or anxiety) symptoms, it is very useful to track their menstrual cycle. When the focus of treatment is a role dispute with a marital partner, you might ask the patient to track arguments with his or her spouse.

During the history taking and the completion of the interpersonal inventory you will ask your patients to begin to complete the SRM-II on a daily basis (see Figure 6.3 for an example of a partially completed short version, Figure 6.4 for an example of a partially completed long version, and Appendices 1 and 3 for blank copies of both versions that you can reproduce for your own use), but will specifically instruct them not to alter their routines until they have a chance to review and discuss the first few weeks of SRM recordings with you, because you will want to have a fairly complete picture of their daily lives before you start to suggest changes. The reason is that a change in one area (e.g., suggesting an earlier wake time) can actually have unintended consequences in another area (e.g., the patient doesn't compensate with an earlier bedtime, becomes sleep deprived, and develops hypomania). These initial SRM records also provide an opportunity to clarify any questions your patient may have about how to complete the SRM. The data gathered on these first SRMs give you considerable information on which to base your case formulation and the specifics of the symptom management plan. If these first SRMs are gathered while the patient is still recovering, additional weeks of data, as the patient becomes more stable, may be required to get a true baseline of your patient's "usual" pattern.

Social Rhythm Metric–II—Five-Item Version (SRM-II-5)

Directions:

- Write the **ideal target time** you would **like** to do these daily activities.
- Record the **time** you actually did the activity each day.
- Record the **people** involved in the activity: 0 = Alone; 1 = Others present; 2 = Others actively involved; 3 = Others very stimulating

Date (week of): <u>Nov. 29</u>

Activity	Target time	Sunday Time	Sunday People	Monday Time	Monday People	Tuesday Time	Tuesday People	Wednesday Time	Wednesday People	Thursday Time	Thursday People	Friday Time	Friday People	Saturday Time	Saturday People
Out of bed	8:00 A.M.	8:30	0	7:45	0										
First contact with other person	8:05	8:30	3	8:00	3										
Start work/school/volunteer/family care	9:30			9:25	3										
Dinner	6:15 P.M.	4:30	2	6:30	2										
To bed	11:30	11:45	1	11:15	1										
Rate MOOD each day from –5 to +5: –5 = very depressed +5 = very elated		–1		0											

FIGURE 6.3. Example of a partially completed SRM-II-5.

Name: _____ Date: __ __/__ __/__ __
                                                    m m   d d   y y

Please Fill This Out at the End of the Day

Day of Week: _____

			PEOPLE						
			0 = Alone						
			1 = Others just present						
			2 = Others actively involved						
			3 = Others very stimulating						
ACTIVITY	TIME	A.M. or P.M.	DAY OF WEEK						
			M	T	W	Th	F	Sa	Su
OUT OF BED	Earlier				1		2		
	Exact earlier time				6:00		6:00		
	7:00		2		2	1			
	7:15			2					
	7:30								
	7:45								
midpoint of your normal range →	8:00	A.M.						2	3
	8:15								
	8:30								
	8:45								
	9:00								
	Later								
	Exact later time								
	Check if did not do								

(cont.)

FIGURE 6.4. Example of partially completed 17-item SRM-II.

| | | | **PEOPLE** 0 = Alone / 1 = Others just present / 2 = Others actively involved / 3 = Others very stimulating | | | | | | |

| | | **A.M.** | **DAY OF WEEK** | | | | | | |
ACTIVITY	**TIME**	**or P.M.**	**M**	**T**	**W**	**Th**	**F**	**Sa**	**Su**
FIRST CONTACT (IN PERSON OR BY PHONE) WITH ANOTHER PERSON	Earlier						2		
	Exact earlier time						6:00		
	7:00		2		2	1			
	7:15			2					
	7:30								
	7:45								
midpoint of your normal range →	8:00	A.M.						2	3
	8:15								
	8:30								
	8:45								
	9:00								
	Later								
	Exact later time								
	Check if did not do								
HAVE MORNING BEVERAGE	Earlier								
	Exact earlier time								
	8:00						0		
	8:15					0			
	8:30		0	1	1				
	8:45								
midpoint of your normal → range	9:00	A.M.						2	2
	9:15								
	9:30								
	9:45								
			10:00						
	Later								
	Exact later time								
	Check if did not do								

(cont.)

FIGURE 6.4. *(continued)*

ACTIVITY	TIME	A.M. or P.M.	PEOPLE 0 = Alone 1 = Others just present 2 = Others actively involved 3 = Others very stimulating						
			DAY OF WEEK						
			M	T	W	Th	F	Sa	Su
HAVE BREAKFAST	Earlier								
	Exact earlier time								
	8:00								
	8:15								
	8:30						0		
	8:45					0			
midpoint of your normal range →	9:00	A.M.	0	1	1			2	2
	9:15								
	9:30								
	9:45								
	10:00								
	Later								
	Exact later time								
	Check if did not do								

FIGURE 6.4. *(continued)*

From the SRM recordings, you should be able to see how rhythmic or chaotic your patient's routines are, whether your patient is typically performing these routines alone or in the presence of others, and, if others are present, whether they are actively engaged with the patient, perhaps even in ways that are not necessarily healthy. This information helps greatly in formulating a plan for symptom management that may either involve efforts to maintain a relatively "rhythmic" *status quo* or efforts to significantly increase the regularity of the patient's routines. It may also involve efforts to increase or decrease the amount of interpersonal stimulation the patient is experiencing.

CASE EXAMPLE

When Candie entered IPSRT treatment, her social rhythms were a mess and her mood reflected it. After her last hospitalization, she had put together a patchwork of jobs—anything to be able to pay her rent. Two days a week, Tuesdays and Thursdays, she had to be up before dawn so that she could open the gym where she worked as a part-time manager and trainer. On Tuesdays and Thursdays, she was done with work at 2:00 P.M. Sometimes she went home and slept for several hours before coming back to the gym to train her evening clients. Sometimes she would just stay and hang out at the gym until they arrived, napping on the sofa in the coffee area if no one was around. The other weekdays she didn't begin work until 4:00 P.M. and had the responsibility of closing the gym. She was supposed to be able to leave by 10:00, but it always took her at least an hour and a half to finish cleaning the bathrooms and the showers. On weekends she worked as the night manager of a pizza shop near her apartment, often not getting home until 3:00 or 4:00 A.M.. Exhausted, but totally wired, she would never be able to fall asleep until 5:00 or 6:00 anyway, so she often went out for breakfast with some of the night crew.

Her IPSRT therapist didn't really need Candie to complete any SRMs at all to know that this schedule had to be a major focus of their work. When she actually saw how chaotic Candie's rhythms were, she was seriously worried about Candie's ability to stay out of the hospital with the life she was leading. A major challenge was convincing Candie, who needed every penny she was earning just to make ends meet, that she had to change her lifestyle if she was going to stay well. Devastated by her hospitalization and devoid of any of her former self-confidence, Candie refused to believe that her college degree would be of any use in finding a regular 9-to-5 job, or that if she found one, she would actually be able to keep it. She was just too insecure right now to budge from the familiar terrain of the gym and the pizza shop. Her therapist decided to begin by trying to consolidate her sleep as much as possible, suggesting that she try to trade her two early mornings with one of the other part-time managers at the gym, or even drop those 2 days and look for a third job part-time job on Tuesdays and Thursday that also started in the late afternoon. Fortunately, when asked, one of the other managers was happy to trade shifts with her. Candie missed seeing some of the early morning crowd at the gym, but her mood improved so markedly within a few weeks that she was convinced that the improvement was worth the change. Now she had a regular wake-up time at about 10:00 A.M. 5 days a week, wasn't napping much during the week, and actually beginning to put her apartment back in order, something she had been completely unable to do since she left the hospital. Next, her therapist focused on getting Candie to give up the Saturday and Sunday morning breakfasts with the pizza shop crowd. By helping her to learn how to keep the social stimulation down a bit while working at the pizza shop (not chatting with every wound-up customer who came in at 2:30 A.M., not discussing Eastern religious philosophy with the guy who ran the ovens), Candie found that she could go right home from work, meditate for a little while, and be asleep by 3:00 A.M. Not great, but a lot better than she had been doing.

Through the use of the Social Rhythm metric, both Candie and her therapist were able to track the improvement in the regularity of her sleep–wake cycle and the extent to which that tended to regularize her other social rhythms, the timing of her meals, entrances and exits from her home, and so forth. They were also able to see how regularizing her routines seemed to be directly related to improvement in her mood and even in her self-confidence. After about a month of very hard work on changing her social rhythms, Candie was even willing to consider updating her resume and thinking about a job search.

Once you have taken the history of your patient's mood disorder and created an illness history timeline, completed the interpersonal inventory, and reviewed the first few weeks of Social Rhythm Metrics, you should be able to make an initial case formulation. This formulation will include a sense of the extent to which various risk factors (social rhythm disturbance, interpersonal stress, medication nonadherence, etc.) have been associated with the onset of each of your patient's mood episodes. Concentrating primarily on the most recent episode, you will decide what weight to give to each of these factors in understanding how that episode developed and what interventions, offered in what order, are most likely to bring about relief from the present episode (if your patient is acutely ill) and protect your patient from future episodes of illness. Is this a person who seems relatively immune to challenges to her circadian system, but very vulnerable in the face of interpersonal stressors? Is this a person who seems to be able to manage the challenges in his interpersonal world fairly well, but becomes ill every time his routine is disrupted? Or is this a person who has never really accepted her illness and whose episodes are mostly associated with discontinuing her pharmacotherapy?

In the first instance, you would probably want to move fairly quickly through the social rhythm work, identify the interpersonal problem area on which you and she want to concentrate, and get to work on that. In the second case, you might spend many weeks stabilizing your patient's social rhythms and only really focus on the minor role disputes with his wife as they affect his social routines. In the third case, you would probably begin with work on grief for the lost healthy self, because until that is done, it is unlikely that your patient will give much energy to stabilizing her social rhythms or to working on an interpersonal problem.

Bipolar disorder is a complicated and chaotic disorder, and IPSRT, because it involves both behavioral and interpersonal interventions, is a somewhat complicated treatment. This makes the initiation of treatment a relatively demanding process and case formulation considerably more complex than, for example, with a patient presenting in a first episode of unipolar depression or panic disorder. Nonetheless, whenever possible, the initial sessions of IPSRT should seem like a conversation between you and your patient, one in which you maintain the empathic stance that characterizes all forms of interpersonal therapy, but one that you structure enough to be certain that all the information you will need for an initial case formulation will be obtained. Appendix 6 is a checklist of what should be accomplished in these initial settings. You may find it useful to clip it to the inside of the patient's chart and review it as you begin each of the first several IPSRT sessions.

SEVEN

Orienting the Patient to Treatment and Individualized Treatment Planning

As should be clear in Chapter 6, the process of orienting your patient to IPSRT and obtaining his or her consent to treatment is a process that begins even before an assessment and history taking.

When we first see a patient who is not in crisis, we give a very general explanation of what IPSRT is and what will happen if the patient agrees to try this treatment. What we say in this explanation depends a great deal on how long the patient has had bipolar illness, what he or she knows about the illness, and what kinds of treatment experiences he or she has had in the past. With patients who have bipolar I disorder, we make clear that IPSRT is intended to be used along with appropriate pharmacotherapy. We describe briefly the evidence for links between interpersonal problems and social rhythm disruption and bipolar disorder episodes. We explain that we will want to learn about the patient's relationships and the day-to-day pattern of his or her life. Once we have that information, together with the patient we formulate a plan for changes in these areas, changes that should lead to symptom improvement and offer some protection against future episodes. If the patient agrees that this seems reasonable, we begin the history-taking process.

As you are creating an illness history timeline with your patient, you are continuing the consent process. You are making the case for the association between social rhythm disruption and illness exacerbations, with the implication that the patient will benefit from working to achieve more stable social rhythms. As you are completing the interpersonal inventory, you are making the case for the relevance of difficulties in interpersonal relationships and changes in interpersonal and social roles to mood symptoms and episodes, with the implication that working to achieve more satisfying relationships and roles will lead to greater mood stability. Thinking back to Jill, whose case is described in Chapter 1 and whose illness history timeline is presented in Chapter 6, you can see how even her earliest mood episodes were related to changes in social routines. During high school, the long days of spring and summer and the absence of a regular routine during summer vacations were consistently associated with a lowering of her mood and energy. When she was in a more consistent routine, she always felt better. In Jill's case, it took the huge hormonal and rhythm disruption associated with the birth of a first child to bring on a full syndromal episode of mania.

What is striking in Jill's case (and common in the histories of patients who receive no psychotherapeutic help for their bipolar disorder until they have been ill for many years), is the high cost of the illness in terms of her personal and professional life. Helping patients to see that high cost and offering the possibility that they can achieve somewhat better control over the illness is one way in which we make the case for all the difficult changes we will be asking them to make and all the hard work we will be asking them to do in the context of IPSRT. Asking a patient like Jill to reflect on what her life would be like today had she not developed bipolar illness can be extremely painful, but it can also be highly motivating to individuals who, like Jill, feel that they have been essentially helpless in the face of this illness. Patients like Jill are fully aware that medication alone does not control their illness and are often greatly relieved to be offered something active they can do to help themselves.

A patient like Tad, who comes to treatment with much less experience of the illness, will be more difficult to convince of the need for any treatment at all, let alone all the changes you are asking him to make in his lifestyle, especially when everyone around him seems to be able to live that lifestyle with no consequences. With young people like Tad, or with older patients experiencing a first episode, your objective is to address their denial that they have the disorder and/or that it will have consequences for them. In such cases, you must use whatever tricks of the trade you have to keep the patient engaged in treatment long enough to break down the denial and long enough for the patient to begin to experience some of the costs of not adhering to treatment, of not attending to the disorder. With patients like this, we tend to "normalize non-adherence," telling them we expect them to not want to take their medicine, to want to drop out of treatment. We simply ask them to tell us about those feelings when they arise and attempt to be as accepting as possible of these feelings, while still reminding them of what the consequences of these choices might be.

Often such patients will terminate prematurely. When we normalize that behavior as well, we find that they will frequently come back to treatment, either when they run into trouble again or when they have had a chance to reflect on how the illness might interfere with achieving their life goals. Some patients, however, are simply not willing or able to engage in the work involved in IPSRT. With such patients, you emphasize the importance of ongoing pharmacotherapy and how much benefit the patient is likely to obtain from medication even in the absence of psychotherapy. Finally, there are patients who are simply not ready to accept any treatment for their bipolar disorder. With these patients, it is important to indicate that you understand their struggle and leave the door open for their return to treatment should they change their minds.

DESCRIBING OTHER TREATMENT APPROACHES

As implied in Chapter 3, you should inform your patient about other approaches to the treatment of bipolar disorder that might be available, including pharmacotherapy alone. If your patient evidences particular interest in one of these other approaches, explore his or her reasons for thinking this might be particularly beneficial. If that treatment is available in your area, you might suggest that the patient meet with a therapist who can provide that treatment and then come to a decision about which approach seems best suited to his or her current needs. If the patient expresses an interest in a marital or family treatment, you might consider whether he or she should be offered both treatments simultaneously. We have experimented with an integrated family and individual approach that combines Miklowitz and Goldstein's family-focused treatment with IPSRT in patients at particularly high risk for relapse, and outcomes were encouraging (see Miklowitz et al., 2003).

DESCRIBING THE TREATMENT PLAN

Once the initial history taking and orientation and consent phase of the treatment is concluded, you then describe your specific plan for the patient's treatment in detail. You explain the dual focus of the treatment on stabilizing social routines and improving interpersonal and social role functioning. You draw on the specific needs you have observed in each of these two areas as you took your patient's history, and offer your ideas about where the interpersonal work might beneficially begin. Depending on the specific case, you might offer two alternative interpersonal problem areas, asking your patient which he or she sees as linked to the onset of the most recent episode. You then describe the way in which the social rhythm and interpersonal aspect of IPSRT will be interwoven throughout the treatment, indicating that you will begin with social rhythm stabilization and move on to focus more on the selected interpersonal problem area while still attending to rhythm stability. Depending on your patient's history, clinical state, and financial resources, you may make a relatively short-term contract for 16–20 sessions, or you may contract for a much longer program of acute, continuation, and maintenance treatment that may last as long as 2 or 3 years. In such cases, you will essentially ask your patient to renew his or her consent as you enter each new phase of treatment. You may well want to involve a family member in the consent process, particularly if your patient is acutely ill or ambivalent about entering treatment. Involving a family member or a close friend in this process has the added advantage of helping that person to understand the kinds of changes you will be asking the patient to make and allowing you an opportunity to explain how the relative or friend can support (or, at least, not interfere with) the work of therapy.

THE INDIVIDUALIZED SYMPTOM MANAGEMENT PLAN

For patients with bipolar I disorder, the symptom management plan will involve both pharmacotherapy and the behavioral interventions focused on rhythm stabilization and mood regulation. The only exceptions to this rule might occur in the case of a woman who is pregnant (and then probably only in the first months of pregnancy) or in the case of someone who has not experienced a manic episode for a great many years. Otherwise, pharmacotherapy seems fundamental to the management of bipolar I disorder. For patients with bipolar II disorder or other less severe forms of the illness, the symptom management plan may simply depend on behavioral interventions.

Pharmacotherapeutic Symptom Management

Current options for pharmacotherapeutic symptom management have been discussed in Chapter 3. Whether or not you are the patient's prescribing physician, you have an important role to play in educating your patient about medication and medication side effects, in observing your patient's response to pharmacotherapy, and in helping him or her to achieve the maximum benefit from it. If you are not the person prescribing, it is important that you establish a collaborative relationship with your patient's prescribing physician. In the ideal circumstance, you and the physician would see the patient together; however, this is clearly not always possible or practical. At a minimum, you should be able to discuss your patient's progress or deterioration with the pharmacotherapist on a frequent basis if your patient's mood is unstable, and you want to be able to contact the physician immediately when you observe marked deterioration or worrisome adverse effects. Most prescribing physicians will welcome your input and be glad that there is a second pair of eyes watching your patient's course. You may, however, encounter the occasional physician who feels you have no right to "interfere" in his or her patient's treatment. In such cases, you will need all your social and diplomacy skills to negotiate for some kind of collaboration in the care of your patient.

In educating your patient about medication, you will review briefly all of the medications available to treat mood episodes and explain briefly what is known about how these medications work. The bulk of the medication education component, however, focuses on the specific medications prescribed for your particular patient. Should the patient's medication regimen be changed at any future point in time, you should provide additional education regarding the patient's new medications. A very important aspect of educating patients about psychotropic medications is education about what the likely time course improvement will be and providing the patient with very specific (and realistic) information about when he or she can expect to return to normal functioning. Finally, you should encourage the patient (and family members) to expect a full remission of his or her symptoms, not simply a response to the medication.

In the case of treatments for mania, you must be certain that the treatment is bringing the manic symptoms under rapid control without leaving your patient oversedated or experiencing other unwanted side effects. With the use of the new atypical neuroleptic medications, this is a reasonable expectation. If your patient begins to experience weight gain (a common side effect of some of these compounds, as well as of lithium and valproic acid), you can suggest ways in which your patient may be able to get this problem under control before it gets out of hand. There is some evidence to suggest that any of the conventional weight control programs (Weight Watchers, Jenny Craig, etc.) can be helpful in this regard. Some of the pharmaceutical companies that make the atypical neuroleptics offer personalized programs free of charge to patients. This is an option you may want to explore with your patient. If your patient is taking one of the older, typical neuroleptics, you must watch carefully for the development of extrapyramidal side effects, as bipolar patients seem to be particularly vulnerable to these problems. Sometimes dose reduction can be helpful in controlling these side effects.

In the treatment of depression, it is likely that your patient will require the addition of an antidepressant to his or her mood stabilizer. Few bipolar depressions can be brought into full remission with lithium or valproic acid alone, *and full remission should be the goal*. Because clinicians are so fearful of the damage a patient can do during mania, many patients are left lingering endlessly in a subsyndromal depression, rather than being treated toward a full and complete remission, which can sometimes look like the beginning of a hypomania. Depression treatment is likely to go much more slowly than treatment of mania. It is reasonable to think in terms of several months before full remission is achieved. Therefore, part of your job is to encourage your patient to be hopeful and patient as long as some improvement is evident. Again, you should inquire about distressing side effects and do whatever you can to help your patient manage these (see Chapter 10 for some suggestions in this regard). If your patient is not improving or side effects are really intolerable, consider a medication change.

Another way in which you can be helpful is in aiding your patient in the process of deciding whether to discontinue antidepressant treatment once his or her depression has remitted. It used to be thought that patients with bipolar I disorder should be treated with antidepressant medications for as short a time as possible because of the concern that these medications might actually induce mania. Now, however, there are several studies (Altshuler et al., 2003; Ketter et al., 2003) suggesting that stopping antidepressant treatment, even after many months of remission, significantly increases the risk of depressive relapse but has no significant effect on the risk of manic relapse. Still, your patient may have unwanted side effects from an antidepressant (particularly sexual dysfunction and weight gain) that figure in the risk:benefit equation.

Another role you can play is in helping your patient to make judicious use of so-called rescue medication, assuming you or your patient's physician is willing to give this kind of medication to your patient or to be available to prescribe it on a few hours notice. We believe that many a manic episode has been averted when a night or two of difficulty in sleeping (or feeling as though there is no need for sleep and recognizing that) has been followed by a few nights of low-dose neuroleptic or benzodiazepine. For a further discussion of the use of rescue medications, see Chapter 10.

Behavioral Symptom Management

During the initial phase of treatment, you will have asked your patient to begin completing one version or another of the Social Rhythm Metric. If your patient is very depressed, very disorganized, or resistant to the idea of "homework," you may begin with the five-item short version of the SRM-II. Otherwise, it is best to start with the longer 17-item version because it will give you a more complete picture of your patient's lifestyle.

Once the patient has completed 3 or 4 weeks of SRMs, you and your patient should review these initial SRMs, looking for those rhythms that seem to be particularly unstable. For example, is the patient going to bed at 10:00 P.M. one night, 2:00 A.M. the next night, and 12:00 midnight the third night? Does there seem to be regularity during the week but extreme deviation on the weekends? If the weekends deviate, does this seem to be in the service of recovery? Are mealtimes regular? Or does the patient seem to be eating only sporadically? Is this because he or she is not hungry or because the patient has not allowed him- or herself the luxury of regular mealtimes? How often does the patient indicate situations in which he or she found "others very stimulating"? Does the patient appear to be able to get to sleep following such interactions?

SELECTING AND CONTRACTING
FOR THE INTERPERSONAL PROBLEM AREA

The other part of the individualized treatment plan is its focus on an interpersonal problem area. The selection of an interpersonal problem area usually depends on deciding which of the IPSRT problem areas is most closely linked to the onset of your patient's current (or most recent) episode of illness. The one exception to this rule of thumb is the choice of the problem we call grief for the lost healthy self. This problem area is typically selected when you are concerned about your patient's level of demoralization about the illness, or about the extent to which distress about and/or denial of the illness will interfere with treatment adherence.

Once you have a clear idea of what the primary interpersonal problem area is, you present this to your patient in easily understandable, nonpejorative terms. After some discussion and, perhaps, some reformulation of the problem as the patient sees it, you and your patient should be able to reach an agreement that this will become the focus of the interpersonal part of the therapy. You will then go on to describe in general terms how you and your patient will proceed to address the problem, what the patient can expect of you in this process, and what you will expect of the patient.

It sometimes happens that although you can clearly see the negative impact of one of these problem areas on your patient's current level of distress, the patient does not see the problem that way. This most often happens in the case of marital role disputes that the patient is unwilling to acknowledge. Rather than enter into a power struggle with the patient over the choice of the focus of treatment—which is likely to result in the patient's dropping out or otherwise not being fully engaged in the treatment process—the wise IPSRT therapist finds a way to reformulate the problem as one that the patient is willing to work on, in the hope that ultimately the treatment may move on to address what the therapist believes is the true source of the patient's difficulty. In the following case example, the patient came to treatment very depressed, and the last person she would have thought to blame for her depression was her husband. Because of the warmth and intensity of her relationship with her mother and sisters, she had not realized how empty her marriage had become. Her emotional needs were being met in her family of origin, until she was separated from them. We suspect, however, that had her therapist immediately suggested marital role disputes as the focus of her treatment, this patient would have dropped out of treatment within a visit or two.

CASE EXAMPLE

Marilyn had recently relocated to the mid-Western city where she was now being seen for treatment of her bipolar depression. Her mood disorder had been in remission for almost a decade, and she was the happily married mother of two elementary school children when her husband accepted a transfer from the small New England town where they had grown up. One of five sisters in a close-knit family, Marilyn had had a built-in social and support network there. She, her mom, and her sisters did almost everything together: shopped, cooked, took their children to soccer games, and went to church. It really didn't matter very much that Mark was hardly ever home. But now it mattered a lot. Marilyn was completely at sea in her new environment. She had a terrible time finding her way around her new hometown, and Mark was always much too busy with his new job to be able to take her anywhere or even take time to give her directions. Furthermore, their second car wasn't dependable, which also hadn't mattered back in New England because there was always her mom's car or one of her sisters' or a brother-in-law who was happy to come and fix whatever was wrong with her car. Within a few months of the move, Marilyn was plunged into a nearly incapacitating depression. She had the good sense to recognize the old symptoms, but not what was going on in her life. Having married her childhood sweetheart, she was unable or unwilling to see how Mark's inattention and thoughtlessness had led to the situation in which she found herself. Whether or not to accept the transfer was something Mark had never discussed with her, nor had he thought at all about what impact the move might have on Marilyn's life—or, more important, on the course of her bipolar disorder. Nor, now that she was in this state, was he able to understand how she had gotten there: She had a beautiful new home in a perfect neighborhood, all the money she could want to fix it up, kids who were thriving, and a husband who loved her. What in the world did she have to be depressed about?

As Marilyn's IPSRT therapist, you would recognize the nonreciprocal nature of role expectations between Marilyn and Mark even though there is no yelling and screaming going on between them. You would also recognize that those nonreciprocal expectations—a role dispute that was well hidden when she was surrounded by the support of her family and didn't need to count on him—are central to the onset of her depression. Finally, however, you would recognize that Marilyn is currently much too fragile to see her situation in this way at the moment, and were you to present a case to her for focusing on the role dispute, it is likely that she would leave therapy. Because your first task is to engage the patient, you will want to think of a way of presenting her situation that will be acceptable to her and will allow you to begin treatment of her depression, with the idea that once she is stronger, you may be able to address the role dispute between Marilyn and Mark. The experienced IPSRT therapist would likely present the problem to Marilyn as a role transition and try to engage her, first, in the challenging process of integration into her new community. Once that was accomplished, it might well be possible to address the aspects of her marriage that had led to the situation in which she found herself and, perhaps, work with both Marilyn and Mark to establish a more reciprocal approach to future problem solving, one that might help to avert subsequent depressions.

How Long Is the IPSRT Treatment Contract?

The length of the IPSRT treatment contract will vary considerably, depending on the form of bipolar disorder from which the patient suffers (I, II, or bipolar disorder NOS), the clinical state of the patient at the time he or she enters treatment, the patient's history of affective illness and, perhaps, his or her family history as well. A patient who is early in his or her illness history but reports a family history consistent with protracted, debilitating depressions or severe, personally damaging manias should definitely be considered for a somewhat longer course of treatment. The patient who is ambivalent about being in treatment in the first place may not be able to help you a great deal in determining what he or she needs in this regard; however, in our experience, motivated patients are often very wise about how much treatment (how frequent and of how long duration) they require. Such patients should have a key role in determining the treatment contract.

The results of our only completed study of IPSRT suggest that motivated patients who receive only an acute course of IPSRT are often able to continue the kind of social rhythm regulation that protects against new episodes on their own, without regular feedback from and the opportunity to problem solve with the therapist. It also appeared that many were able to maintain a balance between rest and activity and adapt to changes in their routines following what might be considered a relatively brief (approximately 16–20 sessions) exposure to IPSRT concepts.

Probably those patients with relatively severe and frequently recurring bipolar I disorder derive the most benefit from a course of treatment that involves weekly acute treatment for 16–24 weeks, followed by a period of bimonthly continuation treatment of 2 or 3 months duration, followed by monthly maintenance treatment lasting at least a year. This gives both you and your patient an opportunity to see how the symptom management plan functions in periods of relative mood stability *and* in periods when symptoms of mania or depression flare up or when a full syndromal recurrence occurs. It also gives the patient an opportunity to practice employing the symptom management plan under your guidance in a variety of clinical states.

In contrast, patients with well-controlled bipolar I disorder or with bipolar II disorder, who enter treatment mainly in the hope of improving already reasonably good interpersonal relationships and social role functioning, and of preventing future episodes, may be able to get all they need from 12–16 sessions of IPSRT. Even if this shorter course of treatment is adopted, however, it is probably best to reduce the frequency of contact toward the end of treatment, with the last sessions scheduled 2–4 weeks apart to allow some additional time for experimentation.

Finally, because bipolar disorder is a lifelong and seemingly ever-changing condition, we always leave the door open for future contact. Indeed, we often contract for just such contact at a specific frequency, such as every 3 or 4 months, after the formal end of treatment. We also try to make certain, when termination is associated with a move to a new location, that the patient has a therapy contact in the area even if additional therapy is not contemplated at the time. The reality of bipolar disorder is that even with careful adherence to an adequate pharmacotherapy regimen, the typical patient will experience many episodes of depression and mania or hypomania during his or her lifetime. A good way to minimize the destruction that such episodes can bring is to have a strong and consistent relationship with a clinician who is ready to restart treatment whenever they occur.

EIGHT

Symptom Management
Stabilizing Social Rhythms and Behavioral Activation

Most of the symptom management interventions in IPSRT are built around the Social Rhythm Metric. Although its most obvious purpose is the regularizing of daily routines, it also serves as a method for addressing the amount of activity your patient is engaged in and the impact of activity on mood. In IPSRT you are interested in guarding against both underactivity and overactivity, depending on your patient's clinical state and the relative frequency of depressions versus manias in his or her history.

In encouraging the patient to make these changes, you will review again the relevance of the circadian system to mood disorders and the relevance of disruptions in circadian routines to the onset and maintenance of mood episodes. The most basic elements of this psychoeducational intervention fall under the rubric of good sleep hygiene and include teaching the patient to establish a regular wake-up time, to avoid caffeine and other stimulants if sleep is disrupted or shortened, to exercise early in the day rather than before bedtime (when exercise can be stimulating rather than sleep inducing), and to create an association between bed and sleep by using the bed only as a place for sleep (not for watching television, doing homework, or reading for extended periods of time).

As you and your patient assess his or her social rhythms, you must determine (to the best of your ability) whether any social rhythm instability observed is a function of symptoms of the disorder or whether the instability reflects self-imposed lifestyle characteristics. Regardless of the causes for the instability of rhythms, it is important to help the patient work toward stabilizing them; however, the rationales behind the importance of regulating them are different. If the rhythm instability is related to symptoms, as is often the case when IPSRT is initiated while the patient is acutely ill, you will argue that working toward stabilizing his or her rhythms can help your patient to manage these symptoms. When, instead, you determine that the major factors in the patient's rhythm instability are self-imposed, you will argue that rhythm instability may be contributing to a less than complete recovery. In either case, you attempt to convince the patient that social rhythm stabilization can have a long-term prophylactic effect, in addition to any immediate benefits of symptom reduction and can help to prolong wellness and improve the patient's functioning during well intervals.

We do not necessarily assume that the typical level of social rhythm stability experienced by patients with mood disorders is different quantitatively from that of individuals without a mood disorder, especially when patients are not in an acute phase of an episode. Rather, we argue that in order to maximize this therapeutic approach, *individuals with bipolar disorder benefit from a higher level of stability than that "required" by persons with no history of affective illness.* Much like a person who suffers from asthma and must alter his environment and behavior in order to protect himself in a way that is not necessary for those without asthma, the person with bipolar disorder will benefit from lifestyle alterations that have little or no value for those without affective disorder.

You then go on to discuss how the rhythm stabilization process will proceed, exploring sources of interpersonal distress that might work against rhythm stabilization, while also identifying persons who are supportive of the patient. You can then discuss the frequency and intensity of your patient's social interactions, other kinds of potential overstimulation, the timing and regularity of sleep, and other social rhythms (e.g., the timing of work), which he or she concludes may be important. By the end of this process, you and your patient should have a tentative, but explicit, plan for beginning the process of change in his or her daily routines, acknowledging the possibility that the plan may need to be revised as therapy proceeds.

An initial, tentative plan for managing this process is laid out in the Social Rhythm Stabilization Schedule (Appendix 7) for the forthcoming week and in the Future Stabilization Goals Chart (Appendix 8). This plan gives the patient a sense of both the most immediate and the more distant goals, as well as some confidence that they are attainable. The patient can then focus on the relatively modest task of, for example, getting out of bed by 9:00 A.M. for the next 7 days, rather than feeling overwhelmed by the seemingly insurmountable goal of preventing any future episodes of mania or depression.

SEARCHING FOR TRIGGERS FOR RHYTHM DISRUPTION

Once the plan for regulating social rhythms has been initiated, you and your patient will review the SRM data and other recent historical information, trying to determine (or at least speculate about) what in this particular patient's life leads to increased or decreased sleep, increased or decreased social stimulation, and so forth. In addition to inputs from the outside (physical and social *zeitgebers*) that may affect the patient's biological rhythms, it is important that you and your patient identify situations, such as concerts, exhibitions, plays, or lectures, in which the patient finds him- or herself becoming overstimulated as a result of internal cognitive, intellectual, or emotional arousal or as a result of excessive social interaction. Once such situations are identified, you and your patient can work to develop strategies for modulating the frequency and intensity of overstimulation in the patient's life.

CASE EXAMPLE

When Tammi, a 42-year-old single female, entered treatment, she was well aware of the relationship between the onset of most of her manic episodes and social and intellectual overstimulation. She was a high-powered saleswoman and almost all of her episodes of mania had followed inspirational sales retreats that she had attended. However, one onset had remained a puzzle to her.

After several weeks of IPSRT she felt she had come to some understanding of how this episode, which had begun on an especially busy workday, was triggered. At that time she was working as a waitress. Having just started her menstrual period, she had not slept well the previous night and was already fatigued when she arrived at work around noontime. The restaurant was a mob scene. She had worked her full 8-hour shift, waiting on approximately twice her usual number of customers in that time, when another waitress called in sick. Her supervisor insisted that she work an additional 4 hours. During this time the restaurant became even more crowded, and the pace more frenzied. At the end of her 12-hour shift, she felt physically exhausted but extremely "revved up," perhaps simply as a result of the large number of people with whom she had had contact, the large number of orders she had needed to remember, and the little tiff with her boss about working the extra hours. She had planned to go to her parents' home a few hours away for the weekend, but when she left work she was just too tired to make the trip. To her surprise, however, when she got back to her apartment she found that she was unable to fall asleep and paced the floor most of the night. By noon the next day, she had been brought to the emergency room by her downstairs neighbors, in a state of manic excitement.

After discussing this incident with her IPSRT therapist, Tammi's understanding in relation to this onset was that the combination of physical stress and excessive social interaction can bring on an episode, even when the interactions are not stimulating at an emotional or intellectual level. A further exploration of this onset led to a discussion of the extent to which the premenstruum and the first 1 or 2 days of menstruation may be a vulnerable time for the onset or exacerbation of any illness, but particularly for the onset of affective illness, and may be a time when patients should be especially careful to avoid any of the triggers of previous episodes.

ACTIVITY VERSUS INACTIVITY

Finding the Right Balance

Although the first parts of this process (developing a plan for rhythm stabilization and searching for triggers of disruption) can be accomplished in a relatively short amount of time, the third and fourth parts of the process (finding a balance and adapting to changes) take long-term experimentation. This aspect of social rhythm stabilization may require many weeks of effort. Using the SRM-II to review activities and interactions, you will try to determine with each patient you treat with IPSRT the amounts of sleep, social interaction, and intellectual stimulation that are associated with the most balanced mood state for the particular individual.

CASE EXAMPLE

Once Jim, a 35-year-old salesman with a 7-year history of bipolar disorder, became aware of the relationship between sleep deprivation and the onset of his episodes of illness, he became highly motivated to monitor his sleep and regulate his activities so that he could prevent any future sleepless nights. During Session 6, he discussed his plans to make a business trip that required about 4 hours of driving in each direction. He noted that in the past he would have thought nothing of such a trip and would have driven both ways in the same day, greatly reducing his sleep the night before his departure—and possibly on his return as well. He then realized that he often had trouble *getting to sleep* after driving home from such a trip. As a result of the emphasis he had now put on regulating his sleep, he decided to divide the trip and stay overnight in a motel. Jim is currently in the process of job hunting, and as he explores various job possibilities, he is keeping in mind the necessity of securing a job that will not leave him vulnerable to sleep deprivation.

One reason that it is imperative that the experimentation in finding the right balance take place over an extended period of time is that seasonal variation in mood often occurs in mood disorder patients and, probably, especially in those with bipolar I disorder. At times, these mood variations may be superimposed on the natural course of affective episodes. Thus, what works well for a patient during the summer may work poorly during the winter and vice versa. It is also the case that in some female patients mood variation related to the menstrual cycle may lead the patient (and you) to believe that a new episode is starting when this is not actually the case. Careful observation of the relationship of mood changes to the menstrual cycle in such patients is essential.

CASE EXAMPLE

Bonnie is a 30-year-old married woman with a 6-year history of bipolar I disorder. She has had three episodes of depression and one episode of mania. After 4 months of IPSRT treatment, it appeared that she was having exacerbations of depressive symptoms during the late luteal phase of her menstrual cycle. After her symptoms were tracked with a daily rating scale over a 2-month period, it became apparent that her mood, energy, interest, motivation, and ability to enjoy things were, indeed, lower during the week prior to her menses. She and her IPSRT therapist have worked on anticipating these monthly changes. Using the SRM, she has lowered her expectations of herself during the premenstrual week. She is cognizant that the amount of pleasure and stimulation she gets from her daily activities and interpersonal relationships will decrease during this "higher-risk" time. In addition, Bonnie, her IPSRT therapist, and her psychiatrist have learned not to make treatment decisions regarding medication changes or changes in their IPSRT approach to symptom management during her premenstrual week.

Although the completion of the SRM and the effort to bring initial stability to the patient's routines is one of the first actual therapeutic tasks in IPSRT, increasing and/or maintaining that stability is emphasized throughout the treatment. Even with patients we have followed for many, many years in prophylactic maintenance treatment, we find that we are constantly reviewing the regularity of the patient's social rhythms, listening for current or upcoming events that might destabilize routines, and problem solving with the patient about how to maintain regularity in the face of the multiple familial, professional, and social factors pulling the patient off schedule.

Maintaining the Balance

Over the course of the first several months of working to define the right amount of sleep, regularity of routines, interpersonal interaction, and so forth, you and the patient begin to learn what kinds of things derail him or her. For example, when the patient plans more activity than can be handled comfortably or without the patient's becoming overstimulated, he or she may find that a few relatively inactive days are needed to recoup energy or to "come down" from his or her excitement. Such recovery days, however, have the potential to lead to the beginning of a downward spiral. Careful assessment of the patient's mood (perhaps by telephone) can help the patient and you determine whether such recovery days are actually beneficial. If so, they can be maintained as a part of the patient's routine following periods of high activity. However, if they seem to lead to an increase in depressive symptoms, you both need to examine more carefully the amount of activity that can be tolerated without requiring recovery and set clear limits in this area. It is essential that both the patient and you keep in mind that this is a lifelong disorder, and it may require many months of experimentation to discover what works best for any individual patient with bipolar disorder.

Important clues in trying to determine what is best before you know the patient well are the relative balance of manic versus depressive episodes the patient has experienced in the past and the relative speed with which each type of episode began. This is information you should have from the illness history timeline. You can turn back to it as your patient's acute episode resolves and the treatment emphasis shifts to prevention of relapse or recurrence.

CASE EXAMPLE

Maria is a 36-year-old separated woman who had been working on the housekeeping staff of a local hospital. When she first entered IPSRT treatment, she was in a severe and protracted depression that had lasted more than 6 months beyond the end of her last mania. It had taken months of work to help Maria make the transition from being a married to a separated woman. Her Catholic faith ruled out the possibility of divorce for her, and she initially saw herself as being in a never-ending limbo with respect to her family and social life. Her IPSRT therapist helped her to successfully navigate the transition to separated status, to reengage with her many other social supports, and to develop a relatively full life. At this point, Maria's therapist returned to the illness history timeline that they had developed when Maria first came into treatment. Her therapist saw that the depression from which she had just emerged was the only significant depression in her 15-year career of bipolar illness. In contrast, Maria had suffered four serious manias prior to the one that preceded this protracted depression. Thus, as Maria became increasingly involved in activities at her church, in reengaging with some of her high school friends, and in developing more social contacts among her coworkers, her therapist now began to watch carefully for signs that Maria was becoming overstimulated and running the risk of another mania. They had extensive discussions about how to spread out her social activities over the course of the week and the month so that no one day or week was too full of activities and that Maria had sufficient "downtime" to counter her natural tendency to become very wrapped up in and excited about things.

With patients who have had many and/or particularly devastating manias, or with those whose ascent into mania generally takes place within a matter of days, the emphasis should be on guarding against too much activity, loss of sleep, or stimulation. With those whose bipolar illness is characterized primarily by episodes of depression, there is probably more leeway in terms of what the patient can tolerate with respect to sleep loss, activity, and stimulation.

When patients are mildly depressed (which many community studies suggest is the baseline condition of the majority of individuals with bipolar illness), however, they may tend to *underfunction* and plan so few activities as to leave themselves without sufficient stimulation or motivation to prevent the descent into a major depressive episode. These patients should be gently helped to see the relationship between a somewhat fuller schedule and improved mood. The SRM, coupled with daily mood ratings, can be of great help in making the case for sufficient and sufficiently enjoyable activity.

CASE EXAMPLE

In many respects Ann's problem was the opposite of that presented by Maria. Terrified of going into yet another mania, of facing yet another hospitalization, and yet another round of ECT treatments, Ann always wanted to keep herself "a little depressed." At 55 she had had enough of manias, and so had her family, which meant that they tended to conspire with her in her desire to remain in a mildly depressed state. The cost of this strategy, however, was that Ann did literally nothing other than move herself from bed to couch to table, back to couch, and back to bed again. A highly intelligent woman with superb social skills, Ann had much more to offer to herself and others than was represented in her current lifestyle. Ann's IPSRT therapist noted that her mood ratings were consistently in the mildly to moderately depressed range and asked Ann what her ideal state would be. On being confronted with this issue, Ann had to admit that she would much prefer to be fully euthymic if she could simply get over her terror of another mania. Using Ann's good understanding of social rhythm principles, her therapist was able to persuade her to try putting a little more activity into her life. Although neither of them thought that going back to the kind of full-time employment she once had was a realistic possibility or a good idea, Ann had almost completely discounted the possibility of any other kinds of activities, but her therapist had not. She encouraged Ann to train as a volunteer at the local children's museum, something that she could do a day or two a week. She also encouraged Ann to reconnect with some of her old friends with whom Ann had had cutoffs during the course of previous manias. Ann found the children's museum work very satisfying but not too stimulating and, to her surprise, discovered that several old friends whom she assumed would never speak to her again were actually quite pleased to hear from her and happy to make arrangements to go out for coffee or lunch with her. After several months of this increased activity level, Ann's therapist pointed out to her that there had been a marked improvement in her daily mood ratings, but no evidence of mania or hypomania. Together they concluded that this level of activity and social engagement was not only safe but might actually have some prophylactic effects, inasmuch as all of Ann's manias had followed immediately upon severe depressions. By guarding against descent into more severe depression through increasing Ann's level of activity and enjoyment in life, both Ann and her therapist concluded that they might be on a path that could help to prevent future manias.

A similar kind of inactivity can be seen in much younger patients, which responds to a similar approach.

CASE EXAMPLE

Stacey was a 20-year-old student who was suffering her first episode of bipolar disorder when she entered IPSRT. She reported having been raised in an upper-class family. Her parents were supportive of her and encouraged her to lead an active life. Stacey had been a high-achieving student who maintained a 3.5 grade point average. She was active in soccer and lacrosse and took a leadership role in several school clubs. Her parents were successful and led active work and home lives. The precipitant of her episode was a transfer from one college to another. She had been at a small liberal arts college where she participated in sports and student government. After her sophomore year, she transferred to a large school and developed a mania, which required hospitalization. Her illness cycled into a severe 6-month depression, and she was unable to return to her college for the spring semester. Stacey reported feeling low, apathetic, bored, and angry at herself for not being able to live up to her family's and her own expectations of herself. She had little energy, low self-esteem, and no interest in engaging in any activity. She was isolated from friends and confused about her worth because of her depression and inability to attend classes, work, and enjoy being around people. Upon beginning treatment, her routine consisted of getting out of bed at 1:00–2:00 P.M., taking 2–3 hours to get her day started (in part because of her symptoms and in part because of medication side effects), and lying on the couch gazing at the television. When her parents returned home at the end of the day, her mood improved slightly because they helped to engage her in some socialization and household chores. She was a little more active on weekends because her parents encouraged her to get up and do things with them. She had insight into the fact that her mood and self-esteem improved when she went on errands or to a restaurant or movie with her parents.

Stacey and her clinician worked on making the connection between her family value of productivity and her low self-esteem. She was able to understand that her poor self-esteem was a result of her inactivity and feelings of uselessness. This perpetuated her depression. Stacey worked with her clinician to structure her time more effectively. Initially, the treatment focused on the timing of her medication and sleep–wake cycle so she could be more functional in the morning. She and her therapist worked on identifying one or two activities she could engage in each day. Because Stacey had been an avid athlete, she chose walking 10 minutes a day, which was increased to 1 hour over a 4-week period. She and her therapist worked on scheduling her walks at a regular time each day. Once she was able to fulfill her walking commitment, Stacey identified volunteering at the Animal Rescue League as a second activity that she thought she might enjoy and be able to manage. The regular volunteering appointments on Mondays, Wednesdays, and Fridays added further structure to her week. Eventually, Stacey was able to build other activities onto these two. She registered and took a class at a local community college in the summer to prepare her for the fall semester at college and began to reengage with some of her high school friends when they returned home in the summer. As she became more productive, her self-esteem, motivation, energy, and interest gradually improved. She began to have more experiences to discuss with her family and friends, which reinforced her progress. Her depression gradually lifted, and she was in a full remission prior to returning to her original college in the fall.

At each session, you should review the SRMs and mood ratings that the patient has completed since his or her last visit in order to assess how stable the patient's routines have been, how active or inactive the patient has been, and what his or her mood ratings have been like. If a patient has not been completing the SRMs or mood ratings, you should take a blank copy of the SRM and attempt to complete such a review in the session, based on the patient's memory, and encourage the patient to return to regular completion of such ratings if it seems clinically indicated.

CASE EXAMPLE

Nancy is a 58-year-old divorced woman with a 34-year history of bipolar disorder. Although the majority of her early episodes were manic, for the decade prior to entering IPSRT she had primarily experienced depressions, with considerable anxiety and occasional agoraphobia. Her day-to-day baseline was in the mildly-to-moderately depressed range. Her social anxiety had led her to severely limit her interpersonal contacts and to do most of her socializing either in her own apartment or in the apartment of one friend who lived nearby. Initially, her therapist focused on getting her to schedule one additional out-of-the-house activity each week. Her therapist then pointed out how much brighter her mood seemed to be on the day before the activity (when she had it to look forward to), on the day of the activity, and on the day after the activity. This led to a discussion of the relationship between out-of-the-house activities and improved mood. Moving quite slowly, the IPSRT therapist then suggested a second activity every other week. When Nancy realized that she could tolerate this without additional anxiety, she and her therapist then agreed on two regular out-of-the-house activities each week. Over the course of several months, Nancy expanded her activity schedule to the point where she was frequently planning social activities for 5 or 6 days each week. Her response to this intervention was a marked improvement in both her mood and her self-esteem.

ADAPTING TO CHANGES IN ROUTINE

Major changes in a patient's routine may be either predictable (e.g., taking a vacation or starting a new job) or entirely unanticipated (e.g., an unexpected firing, a death, or a marital separation). Predictable changes require careful assessment of the various parameters of the change that might be relevant to rhythm stability. In the case of a vacation, you will want to know, How far is the patient planning to travel? Will he or she be traveling across time zones? If so, in which direction? If the vacation involves changing multiple time zones, how will the patient adjust his or her medication? What will the patient's days be like once he or she arrives at his or her destination? Does the vacation involve a full schedule over which the patient has little control, or is he or she free to set his or her own schedule? What kinds of interpersonal stressors, if any, are likely to be involved in the vacation?

In the case of a new job, you will want to know whether the patient's work hours will remain the same or change. Will he or she have to travel farther to get to the new job? Will this job involve more or less out-of-town travel than the previous one? What will the patient's new responsibilities be? Is this position likely to be substantially more, or less, stressful than the previous one? Does he or she have to learn a great deal of new material in order to be competent in the new position—and, if so, how quickly?

In the case of a planned vacation or business trip, you and the patient can plan for ways that the patient can maintain his or her regular sleep schedule and regular pattern of meals and can modulate social interaction in the new environment so that he or she becomes neither bored and lonely nor overstimulated.

CASE EXAMPLE

Even a cursory review of Jill's illness history timeline, which appears in Chapter 1, would suggest how much mood disruption had been associated with taking a vacation. By the time Jill entered IPSRT treatment, she was positively vacation phobic. Yet after a few months of therapy she began to understand why what was supposed to have been good for her spirits so often turned out to be too good and, therefore, disastrous. As she was feeling appreciably better and less fragile, she also recognized how much she would benefit from a change of scenery and a bit of relief from caring for her boys and her home around the clock. Her financial resources were quite limited, but her husband was more than happy to take care of the children and her brother and sister-in-law had offered to send her a ticket to come to Seattle. As much as the idea of a vacation appealed to her, it also terrified her.

When she mentioned the possibility to her IPSRT therapist, he agreed that there were some risks involved, but that if she planned carefully, she might be able to minimize those risks. They discussed what time of day it would be best for her to travel three time zones west (early in the day, so she could avoid being awake much more than her usual 16 hours) and what time of day she should plan to return (pretty much anytime except on the "red-eye"). They talked about whether she would have a room of her own to sleep in (essential) and what kinds of activity, and how much, were planned for her week there. Jill was then able to call her sister-in-law and discuss what it would take to reduce her anxiety about the trip. Not surprisingly, her sister-in-law was willing to do pretty much anything (including sending her own children to sleep at their grandmother's) to make Jill's visit safe and pleasant. They planned an agenda of activities that was interesting to Jill, but modest in scope, and agreed that if it proved too much for her, they would just take a day off and hang out at home.

By putting a lot of effort into the planning of her trip, Jill was able to get some badly needed respite from her regular routine, enjoy the company of people she cared about for the first time in months, and come back refreshed and more confident in her ability to manage her illness.

Because unanticipated life changes of major proportion, such as a death or marital separation, often have much psychological meaning attached to them in addition to representing dramatic alterations in social *zeitgebers*, considerable therapy time needs to be devoted to adapting to such changes. The IPSRT therapist must address *both* the interpersonal and rhythm stability needs of the patient. Having first, of course, demonstrated appropriate empathy and concern for the patient, the IPSRT therapist's initial emphasis is on the maintenance of stability in as many of the patient's social rhythms as possible despite the major role change or loss. This approach may seem callous, but we have found it is actually much appreciated by patients, who report feeling that we have given them an anchor to hang onto in a difficult time. Because working to stabilize social routines is familiar to the patient and is not loaded with emotional meaning, it is usually something they feel competent to attempt even when they are despondent or demoralized by recent events. Once rhythm stability has been addressed, you can focus on the grief and/or role transition work using traditional IPT techniques, while continuing to emphasize the importance of maintaining social rhythm regularity.

CASE EXAMPLE

Stan had been fired from his job as a systems analyst, largely as a result of his mood symptoms, a few months after entering IPSRT treatment. Following a mania that did not negatively affect his work in ways that his superiors were aware of at the time, he switched into a severe and incapacitating depression. Despite the fact that he was in his mid-40s, everyone in his family agreed that it would be best for him to return to living in his parents' home, both for his safety and in order to conserve what little was left of his savings. He found unemployment to be very stressful and became increasingly frustrated, angry, and disappointed, which led to a further lowering of his mood. He yearned for employment not only for financial reasons, but also because it would provide structure, meaning, and satisfaction to his life. His IPSRT therapist has focused on helping him adjust to his unemployment while waiting for his depression to improve. He was no candidate for a job interview at the time.

The initial sessions focused on teaching him the importance of structuring his days and avoiding under- and overstimulation. He and his therapist discussed various ways to structure his life, including helping his mother with regular household tasks, volunteer work, and socializing. Stan was also able to talk about the impact unemployment had on his sense of self and about the kinds of job parameters that would be important to maintaining his health when he is ready to begin a job search.

As you are working with social rhythm regulation, it is important to keep in mind that what may *look* like social rhythm disruption may actually be early signs of a new episode of mania or depression. Did your patient stay up all night to finish a work project because his boss insisted that it be completed by 9:00 A.M. the following day (social rhythm disruption) or because he got so involved in and excited about the project that he completely lost track of time (incipient mania)? Did your patient sleep until noon because her husband was going to be home that day and was happy to make the kids breakfast and get them off to school (social rhythm disruption) or because she was too lethargic and incapacitated to get out of bed and her husband, knowing that, stayed home just to be sure that the children got to school (depression)? In either case, trying to get your patient back on to a regular routine is likely to be beneficial—to prevent new episodes and to ameliorate or short-circuit incipient ones.

BEHAVIORAL ACTIVATION

Behavioral activation has a long and positive history in the treatment of depressions, particularly those of the anergic type. In his first book on depression, Beck (1967) noted the positive effects of behavioral activation on depressed mood and other depressive symptoms. Subsequently, he built behavioral activation into his cognitive therapy for unipolar depression through its emphasis on increasing the number and frequency of activities that are associated with a sense of mastery or pleasure (A. T. Beck et al., 1979). Many years later Jacobson and colleagues (1996) tested the effects of the behavioral activation component of cognitive therapy used *alone*, in comparison with the full cognitive therapy package. To the surprise of many cognitive therapy devotees, they found behavioral activation alone equally efficacious to the complete cognitive therapy package in bringing about a resolution of unipolar depression.

Although the social rhythm monitoring and social rhythm interventions of IPSRT constitute an implicit behavioral activation component (or, more properly, a behavioral activity titration component), once the therapy moves into the preventative maintenance phase of IPSRT and the emphasis is more on the patient's interpersonal life, it is possible to lose sight of the potential value of behavioral activation. Thus, encouraging a patient who had been well, but now appears to be slipping into depression, to evaluate the extent to which there is sufficient activity in his or her life and encouraging that patient to become more active can be a very useful intervention. You may want to go so far as to inquire about your patient's plans for the upcoming week and evaluate his or her expected level of activity. If it seems insufficient (or, in the case of a patient whose mood appears to be escalating, too stimulating), you may want to contract with your patient for specific changes in the week's plan that you believe would be helpful in maintaining or achieving euthymic mood.

Throughout the course of IPSRT, you and the patient work together to maintain the regularity and balance best suited to the management of affective symptoms. However, a number of factors can cause the system to go awry. The question then becomes: To what kinds of changes do you and the patient need to react? Contrary to what may seem on the surface to be the most sensible approach, it is our experience that the dangers lie in underreacting to indicators of depression and overreacting to indicators of hypomania (with the clear exception of markedly reduced sleep) in the majority of patients. This, of course, may not be true for patients who have experienced many episodes of mania and relatively few depressions. In our experience, however, it is imperative that the you and the patient immediately alter the symptom management plan when depressive symptoms appear, whereas it may be safe to ride out mild episodes of hypomania as long as it is clear that the patient is getting sufficient sleep.

NINE

Intervening in Interpersonal Problem Areas

As stated earlier, IPSRT consists of two key components: management of mood symptoms and intervention in the interpersonal problems linked to the onset of the patient's affective episode.

As in IPT for unipolar disorder, the interpersonal interventions are focused on a small number of primary problem areas: *grief*, *grief for the lost healthy self*, *interpersonal role disputes*, *role transitions*, and *interpersonal deficits*. Much of the intermediate phase of IPSRT involves a focus on the interpersonal problem area formulated during the initial phase of IPSRT and agreed upon with the patient. However, you should continuously weave efforts at change in the interpersonal realm together with changes in social rhythms, pointing out how the desired interpersonal changes could have a positive impact on social rhythms and guarding against interpersonal changes that could have a negative impact on social rhythms, or at least strategizing with the patient as to how to minimize the potentially negative impact on routines of any desired interpersonal or social role change.

NORMAL GRIEF AND UNRESOLVED GRIEF

The death of a loved one can be a highly vulnerable time for patients with bipolar disorder. It is both a time of intense sadness and extreme psychological stress and a time when social rhythms are almost always seriously disrupted. Thus, even normal, appropriate grief has the capacity to precipitate new mood episodes in individuals with bipolar disorder. Long before our social rhythm hypothesis was articulated, "funeral parlor mania" was a well-known phenomenon in descriptive psychiatry. Normal grief parallels depressive symptoms such as sadness, disturbed sleep, agitation, decreased concentration, decreased appetite, decreased ability to perform normal activities, and anhedonia. These normal grief symptoms may be extremely frightening for individuals with bipolar disorder to experience. Patients undergoing the grief process may fear that they are in a major episode. It may be hard to determine whether the symptoms represent a grief reaction or a depression. Under the best of circumstances, your support will help the patient undergo the mourning process. Even with your support, however, the psychological and circadian stress may be more than the patient can manage. When that is the case, it is important that the differential diagnosis of depression is made and appropriate intervention (both pharmacologic and psychotherapeutic) is provided as soon as the clinical picture is clear.

If you are treating a patient at the time of a major loss, initially he or she will need help in expressing feelings, learning about the normal process of grief, and allowing the experience of grief. In addition, a large portion of the work should focus on helping the patient keep his or her social rhythms as stable as possible. Bereaved patients will need to keep their sleep consolidated and as regular as possible during this vulnerable time. Through education, support, and exploration of affect, you can be extremely helpful to the bipolar patient during the grief process.

Often patients with bipolar disorder present for treatment having had difficulty in successfully resolving a prior loss. A delayed or unresolved grief reaction may be caused by an anniversary of the death of a loved one, a more recent death, a patient's reaching the age of death of an unmourned loved one, or by the patient's knowing that he or she, or someone he or she knows, has developed an illness similar to that of the deceased loved one. Finally, if the patient was in a manic episode when a loved one died, he or she may have had no opportunity to grieve and may feel quite guilty about not having done so. Furthermore, the patient who was in a manic episode at the time of an important loss may have behaved inappropriately just prior to the death or at the funeral. This, too, can be a source of profound guilt. Sometimes you and/or the patient will be able to connect an episode of illness with a significant loss, but more likely the unresolved grief will not be identified until the interpersonal inventory is completed. It is important to obtain a thorough history of the patient's relationships to his or her deceased relatives and reactions to the deaths. Such factors as inadequate grief or absence of grief; avoidances before or after a loved one died; absence of family or significant others at the time of the death, during the funeral and related activities, and the first few months afterward; impairment of functioning; and onset of manic or depressive symptoms should be explored and discussed thoroughly. These factors can provide clues as to whether the patient is experiencing abnormal or delayed grief. The specific techniques for working with a patient on unresolved grief are described in detail in Klerman and colleagues (1984); however, patients who were manic or hypomanic at the time of the death will probably require additional, specialized interventions related to feelings of guilt about their behavior at that time.

CASE EXAMPLE

Theresa is a 50-year-old widowed mother of three sons, who has a full-time job and lives alone. She has a history of bipolar illness dating from age 18 when she had her first depressive episode. Since that time she has had three manic episodes and two other episodes of depression. Theresa was raised in a strict religious household. She characterizes her parents as having been relatively unsupportive of her. Early on, she turned to the church to seek the support she felt she did not receive from her parents. Although she felt comforted by her religion, she also came to believe that she had to lead a perfect life to be seen as a good woman in the eyes of God. Theresa married a man she met in church and had her first child at the age of 20. In her marriage, she continued to believe that she had to please others to be worthy of their love. Over the course of the marriage, Theresa became mother and father to her children, as her husband gradually became unhappy, withdrawn, and began to drink.

Her last depressive episode occurred in the aftermath of her husband's sudden suicide. Prior to his death, her husband had become even more withdrawn than usual from her and the family. His interactions with them were often negative. He criticized Theresa and their sons, who were now out of the home, for seemingly minor failures. Theresa tended to blame herself not only for all of her supposed failings, but for those of her sons as well. Not surprisingly, just before his death Theresa was making even greater efforts to please her husband. Following his suicide, Theresa quickly readjusted the surface of her life, and to the loss of her husband, but did not show the normal signs of grieving. She resisted the efforts of many friends to comfort her and seemed impervious to her loss until she became severely depressed 6 months later. Theresa described her depression as a collapse into guilt over not having been a good enough wife and mother. Her husband had left no explanation for his suicide, and Theresa filled the vacuum by taking responsibility for his unhappiness. Her previously orderly life began to fall apart as she had trouble staying awake and great difficulty in accomplishing the simplest everyday tasks. Finally, her depressive symptoms interfered to such an extent with her ability to carry out her family and work responsibilities that she needed to be hospitalized.

After her hospitalization and while in IPSRT outpatient therapy, Theresa came to understand that she had been taking responsibility for the feelings of others since she was a small child. Her religious beliefs meshed with her interpersonal style in such a way that Theresa felt enormous guilt for not having been a better wife. Had she been able to make her husband happy, she believed, he might not have killed himself. In questioning this belief in the context of her IPSRT treatment, the guilt that had stood in the way of normal mourning began to resolve. Theresa was able to become angry with her husband for his "abandonment" of the family, first through alcohol and then through suicide. She was also able to become sad over his loss. Throughout the rest of therapy she continued to grieve in a more normal way and worked hard on developing new interests and relationships. She grew closer to her three grown sons and came to see that she had done an excellent job of raising them. She came to feel quite competent in her mother-of-adult-children role. Finally, she was able to use her church as a source of satisfying social activity and social support.

GRIEF FOR THE LOST HEALTHY SELF

After many years of working exclusively with patients who suffered from recurrent unipolar depression, we began a major program involving those with bipolar I disorder. We were immediately struck by the tendency (which we had never observed in the unipolar patients we had treated) of the patients with bipolar disorder to divide their lives in two: before their diagnosis and after their diagnosis. We soon realized that in this new group, a patient often saw him- or herself almost as two different people: the person he or she had been before developing bipolar disorder and the person he or she was now. We began to talk about the idea of grief over the "lost healthy self" as another form of unresolved grief that was common among individuals with bipolar disorder. Some of our colleagues who are experts in IPT for unipolar disorder have argued that this problem area is more appropriately thought of as a subset of the role transition problem area, but we have found that presenting it to patients as a form of grief has a very profound impact and tends to motivate them to work on this issue in a way that presenting it as a role transition does not. Perhaps this is because "becoming bipolar" has a kind of unalterability that is more like a death than the loss of a job or even a divorce.

Many individuals with manic–depressive disease have great difficulty in coping with their illness because of its instability, its bipolarity, and the ramifications of the illness in their lives and the lives of their families. They are often especially frustrated by the limitations the illness puts (or appears to put) on them. Many times, individuals with bipolar disorder experience a real or apparent deterioration in social skills over time. Relationships with family members, spouses, friends, and coworkers are often strained. In the case of Ann in the previous chapter, manic behavior may have resulted in cutoffs with former friends and even with family. As an IPSRT therapist, your task then becomes to help the patient grieve for the healthy self: the self who would be in better control of her moods, would have had the career she had been planning upon entering college, and would have more stable and meaningful relationships with significant others and family.

Patients with bipolar disorder frequently need to compromise their ideals to make certain that their own needs, as determined by their illness, are met. For example, the woman with bipolar disorder who is about to become a mother may not be able to do everything that her idea of the "ideal" mother is able to do and still take good care of herself. A life change such as parenthood often interacts strongly with the desire to deny the illness, even among those patients who have worked hard in prior therapy on various aspects of symptom management. In the case of the new mother, the lost "healthy" self is the woman who would have been able to awaken three or four times a night to nurse a newborn without jeopardizing her health. Once the patient acknowledges that to do so would be to risk another onset of illness, your next task is to help the patient see that "healthy" and "ideal" can be redefined in terms of the exercise of good judgment in caring for herself so that she, in turn, will be capable of caring for the newborn.

CASE EXAMPLE

Ginnie was 38 years old when she became pregnant with her first child. She had suffered from bipolar illness since her mid-teens. She had experienced several severe manias for which she had been treated as both an inpatient and an outpatient. Lithium had always worked well to control her symptoms, and she functioned extremely well when she took her medication; however, she had a history of stopping her lithium every couple of years. When this occurred, she usually experienced an episode of mania or depression that was severe enough to require short-term hospitalization.

When Ginnie was referred for IPSRT treatment, she was almost 3 months pregnant and had not taken any medication for almost 6 months. With her psychiatrist's support, she had suspended her lithium treatment while trying to become pregnant. Things had gone reasonably well for the first 5 months off lithium, but now she was slipping into a depression. Although she had hoped to remain medication-free throughout her pregnancy, her obstetrician, her IPSRT therapist, and her psychiatrist all believed that the period of major risk to the fetus had passed. Even she could see that her clinical condition was deteriorating rapidly. She agreed to restart her medication, and from 3 months gestation to delivery she took her lithium as prescribed. At 40 weeks, she delivered a perfectly healthy 7-pound 5-ounce baby boy.

After the birth of her son, Ginnie had to decide whether to breastfeed her baby, something she thought every good mother should do. Breastfeeding would mean discontinuing her lithium again and waking multiple times each night to feed her son. Although she began this decision-making process very determined to stick to all her ideas of what constituted the ideal mother, when she and her IPSRT therapist went carefully through a systematic analysis of all the pros and cons associated with nursing her baby, she realized that nursing could, in fact, have very negative consequences for her new child. Because, historically, discontinuing her lithium had resulted in Ginnie's experiencing a recurrence of her bipolar illness and the disruption to her sleep involved in nursing added another important risk factor, she decided that it was much more important for her and for her baby to do what she could to maintain a stable mood and stay out of the hospital. What good was it to have the special experiencing of bonding with her child in this way if it meant that she might end up in the hospital, completely separated from him for weeks? With the help of her IPSRT therapist she was able to decide that, for her, being a good mother meant taking her lithium, caring for her bipolar illness, and sacrificing nursing her baby. In fact, at the end of the process it didn't seem like a sacrifice at all. She, her therapist, and her husband worked to find multiple other ways in which she could be close to her new child while remaining on her medication regime and being certain that she was getting adequate sleep.

INTERPERSONAL DISPUTES

Perhaps because a central feature of both hypomania and depression is irritability, and because a characteristic of the "bipolar temperament" is a certain tendency toward an attitude of entitlement, interpersonal disputes tend to be common in this patient population. In our experience, bipolar patients, especially those who are completely independent of their family of origin, appear to have more overt interpersonal disputes with those outside the family than do unipolar patients. Therefore, we include an example of this subset of interpersonal disputes in the following case. Because the same level of understanding and reciprocity cannot be expected from a coworker, a boss, or a neighbor as can be expected from a family member, the strategies you would use in IPSRT to work with a role dispute with a person outside the family may differ somewhat from those you would use in trying to help your patient resolve a dispute with a family member. Interpersonal disputes occurring in the workplace or neighborhood typically require individuals to be more tolerant, patient, and accepting of limitations in themselves and in others. When helped to see that the world is not always a fair or rational place, that changes in relationships frequently take longer than may be desirable, and that superiors are often individuals with limitations themselves, IPSRT patients can frequently learn to restrain their most critical and argumentative instincts, especially when they can be helped to see the negative consequences that such criticism and argument have on their professional advancement, friendships, and even their financial circumstances.

CASE EXAMPLE

Hal was a 29-year-old, single, graduate student when he began IPSRT treatment. He had had a 5-year history of bipolar disorder, with irritability being a prominent feature of both his depressions and his manias. He had great difficulty being stabilized pharmacotherapeutically. He experienced pronounced and distressing side effects when on sufficient medication to control his mood, but became highly irritable and impatient when his medication was reduced sufficiently to diminish its side effects to a tolerable level. He was having considerable difficulty finishing his graduate training. This difficulty resulted both from brief, but incapacitating, acute episodes of illness and from his inability to restrain his critical impulses even when relatively euthymic.

Hal was almost certainly one of the most intelligent students in his graduate program, probably brighter than many of his professors, and therein lay a large part of his problem. He found it difficult to conform to the overall program curriculum and to the specific assignments for papers and research projects, which he frequently characterized as "dumb," even to his professors. Indeed, from the perspective of his IPSRT therapist, he was often technically correct: His program consisted of a rigid curriculum that allowed little flexibility or consideration of a student's past training or experience, and many of the assignments had a distinct "busywork" quality. However, it was equally apparent to this therapist that his litigious stance was earning him nothing but enmity in the program. This was bad enough in and of itself, but it made things especially complicated when he plummeted into episodes of depression. The professors he had ridiculed a month earlier were naturally not as sympathetic as they might have been had Hal been able to keep some of his negative opinions to himself.

In the course of his IPSRT therapy, he came to recognize the extent to which "taking the high ground" was interfering with his ability to finish his degree. Indeed, these attitudinal problems may have contributed even more to his difficulties than the acute exacerbations of his illness. During the two semesters that overlapped with his therapy, Hal was, with constant encouragement and coaching from his IPSRT therapist, generally able to put aside his evaluative instincts and simply complete his assignments. Although his sense of entitlement remained and continued to create occasional problems in certain school situations, he felt he had learned an approach that would enable him to get through the process of proposing his dissertation topic and carrying out his dissertation work without further conflicts with the faculty. Interestingly, his new quieter stance was associated with less variability in his mood. When his therapist pointed this out, Hal had to acknowledge that maybe the emotional costs of these conflicts had been higher than he had realized.

Many young adults with bipolar disorder do, however, experience problems within their nuclear family. Young bipolar patients, often as a result of educational and developmental delays caused by their disorder, are not fully emancipated from their family well after the age at which most of their peers are living fully independently, and do not have age-appropriate relationships with their parents.

CASE EXAMPLE

Lisa came to IPSRT treatment at 19. She had just taken her first job as dental technician and was living on her own in an apartment. She had had several manic and depressed episodes, all of which had seriously interfered with her family and social relationships, as well as with her school performance. Her parents had divorced when she was 6 years old. Although both parents were individually quite devoted to their daughter's welfare, they had only recently been able to work together to help cope with Lisa's mood disorder and interpersonal problems. Perhaps as a result, Lisa typically had had little respect for authority, which was reflected in feelings of moral or professional superiority, especially to teachers, school administrators, coworkers, and her father, whose demands she perceived as evidence of not caring for her or as obstacles to her freedom. This stance has brought her into frequent conflict with others. These conflicts would often intensify when she regarded others' efforts to get her to see their side of things as a form of manipulation. Lisa is quite bright, verbally quick, and technically competent, but she had mostly used her natural talents to avoid the need for compromise. As a result, her relationships and academic record suffered. At the time she presented for treatment, she was having increasing difficulty in getting these old "tricks" to work for her and was struggling to make it financially on her dental assistant's salary. Indeed, although she was very skilled at her work, her boss had already told her that unless she became more consistent in her attendance and more respectful of others in the office, he would need to look for a replacement.

Lisa had long had a pattern of making her needs known to her parents only when she was acutely depressed. At those times, the neediness that was underlying her declarations of independence became quite pronounced and she would tend to pull them in to support her, only to push them away when she felt better. When it looked as though her first job might evaporate, she initiated this cycle once again; however, her IPSRT therapist used it as an opportunity to build a much more mature, reciprocal relationship with her parents. As she progressed in therapy, she became increasingly cognizant of this interpersonal pattern and more aware of how the way she had managed her neediness had left her unfulfilled and even angry with her parents, while also keeping her enmeshed with them in a unnecessarily dependent way. She began to question her view of others' inferiority and to consider her own feelings of inferiority. She was able to explore the disappointment and resentment she felt over her father's leaving the family and began to see the demands he placed on her as concern rather than intrusion. Over the last several months of treatment, the level of conflict with both of her parents diminished, as she was able to define a set of reciprocal expectations with them for their behavior as parents and for her behavior as an independent adult child. She became closer to her father and found that her need to challenge her boss diminished as well. At the time of therapy termination, she was doing well in her job and had formed a long-term relationship with a young man that appeared to be based on mutual affection and support.

Other bipolar patients, who have been functioning well and have been fully independent from family, may deteriorate because of an episode, and consequently, family members may then need to become more involved. Patients may need to become more dependent on them temporarily. Helping patients cope with their dependency and their family members' involvement in their lives can be a major task of IPSRT therapy when this occurs.

CASE EXAMPLE

Walt was a 40-year-old divorced male when he entered IPSRT following his fifth episode of bipolar illness. He had been unemployed for 1 year. During that year he had had a prolonged manic episode, toward the end of which he was hospitalized for several weeks. His wife had insisted on a marital separation early in the mania, and he had lost his job as an electrician with a local construction company. When he was discharged from the hospital, he decided to relocate to his hometown and live temporarily with his parents until he could secure employment and get his personal life back on track. This was a difficult decision for him to make, because he had been living independently for 18 years. From the time he returned, his relationship with his mother was conflictual. His relationship with his father was tense as well. Walt attributed the conflict with his parents to his bipolar illness and his unemployment. Both his parents had difficulty understanding the illness and were inappropriately intrusive, controlling, and protective. They tried to tell him how to live his life and what activities he should do each day. Walt deeply resented this, but felt trapped in his situation. He was actively job hunting, looking for a work as an electrician, but construction work was at a virtual standstill in his parents' small town, and they kept insisting that he look at other careers and broaden his job focus. Because of his illness and because of his age, he felt he needed to remain narrowly focused and not become alarmed about the length of time it was taking him to secure employment.

Walt used the IPSRT therapy to discuss his frustration about living at home and his anger at his parents' intrusiveness and attempts at controlling his life. He was able to recognize that because he was living with his parents and was being supported by his parents financially, there was a tendency for his parents to treat him like a teenager. Understanding that his parents were acting out of concern for him, his illness, and his ability to gain employment helped him to diffuse his anger. His IPSRT therapist and he discussed ways to cope with his parents' intrusiveness. He chose to not react to most of it, but when it became too difficult he tried to set reasonable limits with his parents. When this did not work, he learned to go to visit his sister and distance himself from his parents. In addition, as he learned more, he worked hard to try to educate his parents about bipolar illness. His long-term goal was to have his parents be more involved when he is symptomatic and less involved when he is asymptomatic.

Marital disputes can also occur in bipolar patients. Generally, marriages are threatened in multiple ways by bipolar disorder, and the divorce rate among individuals with bipolar disorder is high.

CASE EXAMPLE

Alex was a 38-year-old married attorney with two small daughters when he entered treatment with his IPSRT clinician. At that time he had a 10-year history of bipolar disorder. His two earliest episodes were depressive episodes, and the last two were episodes of mania. He presented for treatment during his second manic episode only at the insistence of his partners, who were very concerned about his erratic behavior. His symptoms included euphoric mood, decreased need for sleep, talkativeness, increased activity level, increased socialization, increased libido, promiscuity, irritability, and poor judgment, both generally and specifically in his interactions with clients and in the courtroom. His partners were worried that he would be disbarred if something didn't change. His increased socialization and his promiscuity had caused severe martial problems. His wife, who was appropriately suspicious of the late nights out, the phone calls from strange women, and other fairly obvious signs of his infidelity, became unhappy and intrusive. She tried to control his behavior and limit the amount of time he spent away from her and their little girls. The more she demanded of him, the angrier he became. He acted out by increasing the amount of time he spent away from her and the children. Finally, his anger at his wife and his desire for freedom became so strong that he decided to separate from his wife and live independently. They were separated for 8 months. Once the manic episode ended, Alex was able to reflect on his manic symptoms. He regretted his decision to leave his wife and tried to reconcile. However, by this point much damage had been done to the marriage. His wife felt abandoned, betrayed, hurt, and angry at her husband's behavior.

Once his manic symptoms were under control, Alex was deeply upset by the fact that he could have behaved so irrationally and inconsiderately. He needed time to understand how the symptoms had affected his judgment and decision making. He also needed help in figuring out exactly how to discuss this with his wife. If their marriage was to continue, he knew that she would need to learn not to personalize his behavior, despite its profound impact on her self-esteem, but Alex had no idea of how to get her to understand that the person that had inflicted all this pain was not the "real him." His IPSRT therapist suggested two or three sessions with his wife, and she agreed to attend his treatment. During these sessions the therapist attempted to educate Alex's wife about the ways in which mania can affect a person's judgment. At first, she saw the therapist as taking Alex's side. With time and a lot of attention to her side of the story, however, she began to see that Alex's therapist had both their interests at heart, as well as those of their children. The couple decided to reconcile, with the clear knowledge that much damage had been done to their relationship and that much time and effort would be needed to reconstruct the marriage.

ROLE TRANSITIONS

The role transition problem area constitutes one of the truly unique and important contributions of Klerman and colleagues to the treatment of patients with mood disorders. Such transitions can include both apparent losses such as divorce, widowhood, and the departure of children from the household, and apparent gains such as getting one's first full-time job, a major promotion, marriage, and the birth of a child, but both losses and gains require readjustment and change on the part of the person going through the transition. Being generally sensitive to even modest shifts in daily routines, individuals with bipolar disorder can find role transitions to be particularly stressful times.

Role transitions should become the focus of IPSRT treatment when events in the patient's life have caused or are likely to soon cause major changes in the patient's social roles and/or lifestyle. You will want to determine the significance of a change to the patient's interpersonal relationships, social rhythms, and self-image. Clearly, some role transitions will have effects in all three of these areas, whereas others will affect only one or two of them. A role transition can either precede or follow an acute episode of illness, causing or being caused by the episode of depression or mania. Your patients may need help in structuring their lives during a role transition or restructuring their lives following one. You will also want to discuss the patient's feelings about the person and/or role that has been lost and how he or she is managing the new role the patient has voluntarily or involuntarily assumed. Often, patients with bipolar disorder have considerable difficulty in coping with the changes associated with a role transition, especially if it was caused by the bipolar illness itself, inasmuch as guilt, self-blame, recrimination, and bitterness about having the illness can complicate the role transition work. Sometimes the role transition will provoke shame and/or a sense of humiliation, thus deeply affecting self-image. This can be particularly true when symptoms of mania or depression lead to a person's being asked to leave school or college, employment termination, eviction, or separation or divorce. Often, in the context of such losses, a mature person who has been living independently for years is forced to return to the parental home and becomes, once again, dependent on his or her parents. This kind of transition can dramatically and rapidly lower the patient's self-esteem.

CASE EXAMPLE

Melissa was a 38-year-old married woman who was raised in a stable family environment. She was very close to her family of origin and identified her three sisters as constituting her primary social network. She was also extremely close to her mother, who had a major influence on her life decisions and self-esteem. Her mother was extremely proud of her. Melissa reported having a stable marriage and three children, a 10-year-old and 5-year-old twins. She worked as a nurse and considered herself an excellent mother, wife, and employee. She reported having a mildly hypomanic baseline until the birth of her twins. At that time she had a mild postpartum depression and then experienced her first mania approximately 3 years after their birth. Since her mania 2 years ago, her mood had been cycling and had not stabilized at the time she began IPSRT. She continued to work full time but admitted that her work had compromised her other roles. Her illness and inability to function as well as she had in the past represented increasing sources of frustration. She had prided herself on her strength, ability to raise a family, have a career, and attend to her mother's and sisters' needs. Because her moods were rapidly cycling, she was unable to rely on herself. Her interpersonal relationships were conflictual because she would either be disengaged from her immediate family or overinvolved with them and overscheduling activities for them. She had a great deal of difficulty in accepting her bipolar illness and the way in which it was affecting her interpersonal functioning. After discussing all of these changes with her therapist, she had to give up the "healthy" role in the family and face the implications that would have. The treatment focused on helping Melissa assess her roles as wife, mother, daughter, and nurse in light of her bipolar disorder. She gradually accepted that she would not be able to engage in all these roles at the level she had maintained prior to her mania. Much of the therapeutic work focused on helping her decrease her expectations of herself, sacrifice some roles or change her perception of how to perform in those roles, and learn how to take better care of herself. She decided to work part time in a doctor's office rather than in a stressful inpatient hospital setting, develop some distance in her close relationship with her mother, allow her sisters to help when she could not, and allow her family to help her when her mood was unstable. She had to work hard on changing her self-perception of being the "supermom" in order to do this. Melissa and her therapist continue to work on coping with the bipolar diagnosis, making adaptations in her life in order to manage her moods and roles more effectively.

Almost all patients with bipolar disorder will experience role transitions as a consequence of their illness. Some patients are able to accept them and are eventually able to return to their pre-episode functioning with little or no impairment once the episode resolves. Some bipolar patients will have more permanent changes or impairments as a result of their illness. Still others will appear to weather the storm of their first several episodes with no clear diminution in role functioning and then later show a pattern of social role deterioration as the episodes, hospitalizations, job losses, and residential displacement that are often associated with severe episodes, accumulate. The patient who was able to return to her job 3 days after each of her episodes in her 30s, may be unable to do so a decade later and find herself in markedly reduced circumstances or even homeless by the time she reaches her late 40s. The consequences of manic symptoms, such as poor judgment, promiscuity, spending sprees, irritability, grandiosity, and impaired decision making, may be devastating to patients' lives. Any of these symptoms may lead to unplanned and undesirable role transitions.

CASE EXAMPLE

Pat was a 52-year-old divorced former secretary with a 30-year history of bipolar disorder who entered IPSRT following a severe mania that cycled into depression. During an earlier episode, which occurred after discontinuing her prescribed medications, she experienced expansive mood, inflated self-confidence, a need for less sleep, increased energy, decreased appetite (often forgetting to eat), racing thoughts, and poor judgment, especially apparent at work. She was acutely embarrassed by her behavior. At the time, she had been working at the same company for 5 years. She quit her job, even though her employer was willing to take her back, and then held several short-term jobs for various other companies, but was never quite able to make ends meet again. Always religiously oriented, she turned to her faith for consolation. Imperceptibly, what had been normal religious devotions turned to hyperreligiosity. Pat began to interpret events and occurrences as messages sent from God. Through her church, she met a man who had multiple psychiatric problems and a history of frequent inpatient hospitalizations. Pat was convinced that God had sent this man for her to "save." She withdrew $8,000 from her IRA account and charged $5,000 on her credit cards to take care of him. Unable to pay her bills, she was thrown out of her apartment during her mania and was forced to relocate to an apartment in a very undesirable area.

Once her mania remitted, Pat found herself in a depression unlike any she had experienced in her 30 years of illness. Pat's therapist was challenged to help her cope with the multiple unpleasant changes brought about by her illness. She was very unhappy with her apartment and neighborhood, but was unable to move to a better place because of the financial predicament her most recent manic episode had caused. She had previously been reasonably successful and well paid as a secretary, but was now able to find work only as a phone solicitor. She had many debts and no clear means of extricating herself from them. She had severed many of her friendships during her period of hyperreligiosity and now was quite socially isolated. She was terribly discouraged by the transitions that had occurred in her life, and in the first part of her role transition work, her IPSRT therapist concentrated on helping Pat to grieve her many losses.

Not convinced that Pat was actually capable of returning to the kind of high-level secretarial work she had done before, her IPSRT therapist decided to concentrate on helping Pat to rebuild her social network. To her surprise, many of her old friends were pleased when she recontacted them and happy to spend time with her again, even if she could not afford some of the activities they had shared in the past. This led to a marked improvement in her mood. Her therapist then encouraged her to seek some professional financial advice about how to reduce her debts. She learned that she could declare personal bankruptcy, and even though this did not lead to any marked change in her living circumstances, it did mean that she experienced far less guilt about not being able to pay off all of her debts. Although Pat will probably never return to the level of role functioning she had experienced previously, she completed her acute IPSRT therapy much less depressed and more accepting of her circumstances. In her maintenance treatment, Pat's therapist will focus on preventing further deterioration in her work functioning, will continue to encourage her socialization with old friends, and will monitor her involvement with her church and her religion to be certain that it remains rational.

As implied in the section on the management of affective symptoms in Chapter 8, role transitions in IPSRT require considerably more integration with symptom management than in the case of IPT for unipolar disorder. In the best of circumstances, role transitions are planned or at least anticipated. You can help your patients to acknowledge in the planning that the disorder may set limits on the extent to which they can conform to the new role expectations. In IPSRT adjusting to the demands of a new role interacts constantly with the management of affective symptoms.

CASE EXAMPLE

Jenna was a 19-year-old college sophomore with a 5-year history of mood episodes when she was referred for treatment by the university counseling service. Because of her affective illness Jenna had begun college in her hometown. She continued to live in her parental home throughout her first year of college. Her freshman year thus seemed little different from high school. At the end of her freshman year, she and her parents agreed that she was ready to try going to school away from home. This role transition proved much more problematic than either she or her parents could have imagined.

Released from the routine of her parents' home and free to plan her class schedule within the framework of a large university (as compared with the small college she had been attending near home), Jenna found herself in deep trouble, both academically and symptomatically, within a few months of beginning her sophomore year. Although she loved the freedom of the dormitory and the ability to set her schedule so that none of her classes began before noon, with a little exploration she and her IPSRT therapist were able to see how her sleeping in tended to promote her depressions and prevented her from studying in the early to mid-morning, formerly her productive time.

After several meetings with Jenna's frantic parents, her therapist was able to clarify the fact that the problem was not so much in her new role as emancipated young adult as in the choices she had made with respect to when to schedule classes and when to plan to study. Without changing her first semester class schedule, it was possible to make some adjustments in her sleep–wake and study times so as to provide her with an opportunity to study at her most productive time. This resulted in some improvement in her grades and considerable improvement in her mood. The real change, however, occurred during the second semester when she chose a schedule that was conducive to optimum mood and optimum capacity for study. At the end of her sophomore year, both Jenna and her parents were extremely pleased with her ability to maintain her emancipated status and her euthymic mood.

Often it is your task as an IPSRT therapist to help your patient come to terms with the limitations the illness places on his or her ability to perform certain roles. At times patients may need to rethink their choices of social and work roles and make some changes to decrease stress and overstimulation. IPSRT can help the patient to grieve for the role he or she needed to give up, look at the benefits of not having that role, and make a smooth transition to a new role.

CASE EXAMPLE

Katie was a 41-year-old married woman who had had a successful career as a bank executive. For most of the 12 years she had had bipolar disorder, she had suffered from discrete and relatively brief episodes of the illness. When she entered IPSRT, her moods had been cycling for the past 1½ years and she had been on disability leave for more than a year. Within a few months of beginning work on her social rhythms, she was able to achieve a 2-month period of stable mood and was preparing to return to her job. Unexpectedly, her mood cycled down again, and she knew she would be unable to return to work at that time. She was offered the opportunity to be laid off with severance pay. After a very painful decision analysis with her therapist, she decided to terminate her employment and become a full-time homemaker.

Her IPSRT therapist and she have worked on coping with the grief associated with not returning to work, the loss of that role, and loss of the relationships she had had with her coworkers. In addition, her therapy focused on helping her to see the positive aspects of not working. These included relief from the pressure of having to work, while coping with the uncertainty of whether she would be able to function on the job with her mood swings, and being able to do all the "mom" things she had never been able to do while working full time. As she came to accept her decision, she was able to get pleasure and satisfaction from her new role and to develop a new circle of friends with similar life roles. Her children were delighted with their new mom, and their pleasure improved Katie's mood and helped her to feel more certain that she had made a good decision. IPSRT helped her make a smooth transition to full-time mother and homemaker. Eventually she was able to acknowledge that the pressure of being a career woman, coupled with caring for three children, was too stressful for her and had probably played a key role in her long period of symptomatic instability. Economically, life was definitely more of a challenge, but she and her husband concluded that altogether the family was functioning much better.

INTERPERSONAL DEFICITS

The interpersonal deficits problem area clearly presents some of the greatest challenges for the IPSRT therapist. Because interpersonal deficits tend to be a more pervasive and, at the same time, more amorphous problem in the patient's life, it can be more difficult for you to conceptualize and treat a deficits case than a clearly defined role dispute or role transition. Therefore, we often choose to do interpersonal deficits work later in treatment; this is a problem area we try to avoid as the initial focus of IPSRT unless there appears to be no other interpersonal problem area related to the onset of the patient's most recent episode.

The interpersonal deficits seen in patients with bipolar disorder typically fall into the category of the "chronically dissatisfied" type, who often have disputes with almost every important person in their lives or those who find themselves in self-imposed isolation following a mania that has made them wary of social contact. In our experience, bipolar patients rarely exhibit the chronically socially isolated form of interpersonal deficit frequently observed among unipolar patients, *unless* the patients have managed to alienate most of their social contacts during prior episodes. More typically, the lives of bipolar patients with interpersonal deficits are characterized by numerous, but largely unsatisfying relationships. This is often the result of patients' irritability and their tendency to either idealize or vilify others, with a strikingly absent capacity for accepting both the good and bad in others. Often, this leads to work that consists of what might be thought of as a whole series of individual role disputes, in which you try to help the patient to see the thread or threads connecting the multiple disputes in his or her life.

CASE EXAMPLE

Meredith is a 30-year-old single female who has worked on and off in travel agencies since graduating from high school. In Meredith's case, her interpersonal deficits interacted strongly with the need for symptom management, particularly in the area of social stimulation. Meredith had worked both in isolated settings and in large offices. When working alone, she had a tendency to feel understimulated and to put off taking care of details that needed attention. Yet when she worked in an office with many coworkers, her pattern was immediately to divide her coworkers into the "good" and "bad" groups. Both groups, however, produced problems for her. She was attracted to the "good" coworkers as companions, enjoyed spending time with them and socializing with them, but often found that she became so overstimulated in their company that she was unable to concentrate on her work and sometimes was unable to fall asleep when she got home after a night on the town with them. The "bad" coworkers irritated her with their inefficiency, lack of attention to detail, and "stupidity." Often she became preoccupied with their failings to the point that she could not concentrate on her own work.

IPSRT therapy focused first on helping her to see both groups of coworkers in a more balanced way, to recognize that some members of the "good" group also occasionally failed to pay attention to details or get things done. Moreover, there were positive things about each of the members of the so-called "bad" group. When probed, Meredith was able to acknowledge that the performance differences were not nearly so great in reality as they were in her imagination. She was eventually able to put some limits on her rumination about the performance of the "bad" colleagues, even to see some of their deficits as similar to her own and, most important, to concentrate on her own work. She and her therapist then began working on setting some limits on her interaction with her more appealing coworkers, limiting the number of days each week that she went out to lunch or engaged in after-work social activities with them. Although she missed the fuller social life that she had enjoyed before, she acknowledged that her mood became increasingly stable as a result. She also expected that her annual performance evaluation would reflect her improved work performance.

The socially isolated patient with bipolar disorder, as noted earlier, is generally not someone without social skills. Among unipolar patients we do see those who have never had many social contacts, are extremely uncomfortable in almost all social situations, and have been so since childhood. More commonly, the bipolar patient with the socially isolated form of interpersonal deficit is someone who has burnt his or her social bridges.

CASE EXAMPLE

Steve, the 50-year-old government worker described in Chapter 6, presented with the socially isolated form of interpersonal deficit. When he entered treatment, he had relocated from the city where he had been living and working, to his mother's home in the town in which he grew up so that she could care for him following his hospitalization for a very severe mania. His mother and his sister were the only people with whom he had any social contact beyond the "How's it goin?" he exchanged with the young guys at the gym he now frequented. He didn't even know their names. His shame over what had happened to him and his career left him too embarrassed to contact any of his old high school friends, many of whom still lived in the area. Indeed, if he saw one of them on the street he would try to avoid having to speak to them. He thought about going back to the city where he had worked, but was afraid that no one there would speak to him after the awful things he had said to them while manic—and he was probably remembering only half of it! Steve's therapist worked with him on building a small circle of people his age with whom he could socialize, beginning with a few friends of his brother and sister-in-law's who knew the story of his illness and seemed understanding. His therapist also used the therapeutic relationship to remind Steve of what an interesting person he was, how many things he knew about, and how pleasant it was to converse with him when his mood was normal. This gave Steve the confidence to make contact with a few selected old friends of his own and to begin to think about looking for work again.

The preceding case examples are snapshots of instances occurring in the course of longer-term treatments in which multiple interpersonal problem areas were typically addressed over the course of therapy. Most of our IPSRT experience has been with patients who entered treatment during an acute episode of mania or depression and who remained in treatment for 2–3 years. During that time, some experienced new episodes of illness. In those cases, the focus of treatment returned to an emphasis on stabilizing social rhythms and to whatever interpersonal problem area seemed most related to the onset of the new episode. Among those who remained well following their initial episodes, much of the focus of their preventative maintenance treatment was anticipatory: How can we avoid letting this anticipated loss or change lead to another episode, or how can we prevent this small disagreement from becoming a major role dispute? As an IPSRT clinician, you will want to adjust your work on interpersonal problem areas to the expected duration of each patient's treatment and to the needs that arise as the patient's life unfolds during therapy.

Although termination work is a focus of most of the empirically supported short-term interventions for mood and anxiety disorders, we argue that this needs to take a somewhat different form with individuals who suffer from what is, in almost all cases, a lifelong illness. This topic is addressed in Chapter 14.

TEN

Intervening
Other Useful Interventions

In addition to the two major components of IPSRT, management of mood symptoms through social rhythm interventions and interventions in the interpersonal arena, a number of other interventions can support the overall IPSRT model and can be useful either in the improvement of acute mood symptoms or in the maintenance of stable mood. This chapter describes interventions that we have found particularly useful in employing the IPSRT model for patients with bipolar disorder. The first five are interventions we use with all IPSRT patients. The rest are interventions we have used when appropriate. Therapists who understand bipolar disorder well and are clear about the case formulation can undoubtedly generate many additional creative interventions that fit well with the IPSRT model.

ESTABLISHING A "RESCUE" PROTOCOL

Because the clinical condition of individuals with bipolar disorder can deteriorate very rapidly, it is important that patients and family members agree to a rescue protocol while the patient is in a euthymic state. Such rescue protocols can involve a number of different kinds of interventions. One intervention that we have found to be extremely helpful involves the availability of a small amount of antipsychotic medication to be used to induce sleep at any time a patient finds that he or she is having difficulty in getting to sleep for more than one or two nights and, in highly vulnerable patients, when they are unable to get to sleep after more than a few hours. Consistent with our emphasis on circadian instability and its role in the onset of new episodes of bipolar illness, we believe that one or two nights of missed sleep can be sufficient to trigger a mania.

The relationship between lost sleep and the onset of mania is often confusing to patients and families in that lack of sleep can be a symptom of mania, but inability to sleep can come from a number of causes and, in turn, lead to a mania. Whatever the source of the insomnia (incipient mania or some external influence), the bottom line is that restoring sleep appears to have a clear antimanic effect. We believe that many of the patients in our care have been spared full-blown episodes of mania through the availability of rescue neuroleptic medication. We generally recommend that a patient contact his or her clinician or a member of the treatment team before initiating the use of such medication; however, we strongly recommended the use of the rescue medication (and contact with the clinician on the following day) when the patient is unable to contact the clinician at the time the medication appears necessary.

Rescue protocols may also involve specific and even signed agreements between the patient and family members or significant others as to what each will do (in addition to the use of rescue medication) when the patient's mood appears to be escalating or slipping, but the patient is unwilling or unable to do anything about it. Such protocols may involve permission for a family member to contact the patient's clinician, permission to involve other family members in attempting to help the patient to see that his or her mood is markedly changed, or permission to transport the patient to a psychiatric emergency room or even to request an involuntary hospitalization.

MEDICATION MONITORING

As implied in Chapter 2, medication treatment appears to be essential for individuals suffering from bipolar I disorder in all but the most exceptional circumstances. As indicated in the case example of Ginnie in Chapter 9, women wishing to become pregnant or to carry a baby may be able to go without medication for brief periods of 3–6 months without adverse consequences to their moods; however, it is the rare patient with a bipolar I disorder who can manage for periods much longer than that, and many patients become symptomatic within days or weeks of stopping their medication. Furthermore, unlike patients with recurrent unipolar disorder, who frequently seem to be able to achieve long periods of stable mood by remaining on the same dose of medication, our experience suggests that many patients with bipolar I disorder require fairly frequent adjustment of their medication doses in *either* the upward or downward direction, as well as occasional to frequent changes in their entire drug regimens. Some patients with bipolar II disorder may be able to achieve and maintain stable mood with IPSRT alone, but medication should always be considered as a potential treatment option when IPSRT alone seems insufficient.

Often, as an IPSRT therapist, you will be seeing a given patient much more frequently than his pharmacotherapist and will be able to observe subtle changes in your patient's mood and functioning. In this case, a part of your responsibility is to monitor the extent to which the patient's medication seems to be doing its job. This is not to say that medications should be adjusted with every tiny shift in mood, but to imply that clear changes in mood or functioning that persist for more than a couple of weeks should be a signal to consider a change in the patient's medication regimen. If you are also the patient's pharmacotherapist, you can make this adjustment yourself. If, however, your patient's medication is being prescribed by another clinician, you will either want to consult with your patient's pharmacotherapist yourself regarding the changes you have observed and your concern that a change in medication may be indicated or, even better, help to direct your patient as to how he or she can make clear to the pharmacotherapist the kinds of changes that have occurred. For some of the medications used in the treatment of bipolar disorder, most especially lithium, the patient's blood levels can be an important guide to medication adjustment. Blood levels should be monitored, at a minimum, every 3 months. Even if you are not the patient's pharmacotherapist, it is important that you know what these levels are, as they can indicate a possible change in the patient's adherence to treatment (which can in turn be a sign of hypomania) or a change in the patient's physiology. Unfortunately, some of the newer medications, like lamotrigine, that are used quite effectively to treat bipolar depression show no clear relationship between blood level and therapeutic effect that can be used to guide the clinician. If your patient is being maintained on one of these medications, you will want to inquire about the regularity with which he or she is taking the medication and about any changes observed in the effect of the drug.

SIDE EFFECT MONITORING AND MANAGEMENT

A key component of the successful treatment of patients with bipolar disorder is the review and management of all common side effects (including weight gain and sexual dysfunction) of the medications being used by a patient at each treatment visit. Each potential side effect should be inquired about *directly*, rather than waiting for spontaneous reports of distress by the patient. Even nonphysician clinicians should address the issue of somatic complaints that may be related to the medication the patient is taking, because distressing side effects are probably the second most important reason, after denial of the illness, for nonadherence. Unless you are fully aware of what may be bothering your patients in the way of side effects, you may have a difficult time helping them to accommodate to them or to suggest strategies for actually treating them as well.

None of the medications used to treat bipolar disorder is entirely benign. All carry some side effect burden for most patients. Understanding the nature of the side effects your patient is experiencing and trying to provide help in managing them can greatly improve the chances that your patient will adhere to his or her treatment regimen. Lithium, for example, is associated with polyuria (excess production of urine), which can lead to problems with incontinence, especially in cold weather. You may be able to help your patients manage this by problem solving with them about strategies to reduce the amount of urine in the bladder at any given time and to minimize their exposure to the cold. Lithium can also produce diarrhea in some patients, but this can often be ameliorated through dietary change, as can the constipation that is associated with some of the older antidepressant drugs. A patient can carry a bottle of water or chewing gum to relieve the dry mouth that often goes along with these drugs. You may want to keep a series of one-page handouts for your patients about dietary management of such problems.

Many of the SSRI antidepressants produce nausea, especially early in treatment. Keeping the stomach full, through eating multiple small meals throughout the day, can help, and some patients find that anti-seasickness wristbands alleviate the symptoms. Probably more important than whether any of these interventions actually reduce the unpleasant side effects your patient is experiencing, is the evidence of your concern when you take time to inquire about and offer suggestions for management of uncomfortable side effects.

When side effects are severe and unresponsive to both medical and behavioral management, you or you and the patient's physician should consider alternative treatment and discuss alternative treatment possibilities with your patient. Any decision to change the treatment regimen is made collaboratively with the patient because, in our experience, even patients who are experiencing a reasonable level of distress from a particular side effect may be unwilling to change their medication because the improvement in clinical symptoms has been sufficiently remarkable.

CAREFUL REVIEW OF CONSUMPTION OF OTHER MEDICATIONS, ALCOHOL, AND ILLICIT DRUGS

Your inquiry about somatic distress should also include questions about any prescribed over-the-counter medications, herbal preparations, illicit drugs, and alcohol that the patient has used since the last clinic visit. This is done for two reasons. First, it can be helpful in understanding why a patient who was formerly free of distress from somatic symptoms might now be experiencing them and to be sure that your patient is not consuming anything that could lead to a potentially dangerous drug–drug interaction. Second, patients with bipolar disorder have a strong proclivity for any substances of abuse that temporarily relieve distress, boredom, anxiety, etc.; these often in the end have a very negative impact on the course of their disorder.

We have tended to take a strong negative stance with respect to consumption of alcohol and other mind-altering substances in all patients with mood disorders. Although we don't expect patients to abstain *completely* from alcohol (Of course, you can have a glass of champagne at your niece's wedding!), we do remind patients *constantly* that alcohol has nasty effects on mood when one is on the descending arm of the blood alcohol curve. It has equally nasty effects on sleep, robbing one of the restorative deep or delta sleep that patients with mood disorders are already short on. With respect to illicit drugs, although we make it clear that we understand perfectly well why individuals with mood disorders might be attracted to a wide range of mind- (and energy-) altering substances, we make a very strong case that using them—even in small amounts on an occasional basis—really serves to *undo* all the hard work the patient is putting into stabilizing his or her mood, energy, sleep, and functioning.

In addition to establishing a rescue protocol to be used when new episodes occur, monitoring medications and side effects, and monitoring the use of other medications and substance use, with some patients you may find it important to discuss their nutrition and exercise, address the seasonal pattern of their illness, involve their family members in the treatment effort, help them access a support group, and provide certain kinds of instrumental support. Each of these useful interventions is discussed in the following sections.

EXERCISE AND NUTRITION CONSULTATION

Although patients with bipolar disorder are apparently no more likely to be overweight or obese than persons in the general U.S. population, overweight/obesity is a correlate of poor outcome of the disorder (Fagiolini, Kupfer, Houck, Novick, & Frank, 2003). To make matters worse, many of the medications used to treat bipolar illness tend to produce weight gain. However, it has been our experience that patients who participate in exercise programs and dietary restriction can realize the same benefits as persons in the general population. This means that you have a responsibility to encourage your patients to maintain a body mass index within the normal range (<25). Specific suggestions as to how they can do this are appropriate when patients are motivated to make such changes. We have found that sensible, gradual weight loss programs (as opposed to fad diets), such as those proposed by Weight Watchers, are associated with good outcomes when the patient adheres to the program, even in patients who must continue to take medications that usually lead to weight gain. Regular aerobic exercise, combined with caloric restriction, will produce the best results and may also have mild mood-elevating effects. Such exercise need not be strenuous. Even 20–30 minutes a day of brisk walking can be beneficial. Strenuous aerobic exercise, however, such as long-distance running, may aid some patients in the control of their hypomania. A regular program of exercise can provide an important anchor in the establishment of regular social rhythms and can have multiple health benefits, improving physical health as well as stabilizing mood. For patients in whom the problem of weight gain is severe, consultation with a professional dietician and/or exercise physiologist may be indicated.

MANIPULATION OF LIGHT

A somewhat trickier intervention to aid in the regularizing of social and even true (internal) circadian rhythms is the manipulation of available light. Light, of course, has clear effects on the circadian system, and bright light treatment is used by itself as an intervention for seasonal affective disorder.

In fact, many patients with bipolar disorder have a clear seasonal component to their illness, with spring and summer being associated with mania or hypomania and winter being associated with depression. The use of the high-intensity artificial light boxes used in the treatment of classic seasonal affective disorder is probably not recommended in patients with bipolar I disorder because of the risk of inducing mania. For patients with bipolar II disorder, however, high-intensity light can generally be a safe and effective intervention that provides a remarkable amount of relief of depression symptoms and aids in establishing a more normal sleep–wake cycle. This, in turn, makes all other aspects of social rhythm stabilization easier.

For patients with bipolar I disorder, you may want to suggest, after consultation with the patient's pharmacotherapist, that the patient extend his or her exposure to *natural* light by rising early and getting as much exposure to sunlight as possible. Even this, however, should be done with caution and carefully monitored.

INVOLVING FAMILY MEMBERS

A very useful intervention in the treatment of almost all patients with bipolar disorder is the involvement of family members. In the context of IPSRT, this involvement may be limited to simply educating the family member about bipolar disorder and offering some nonspecific support related to your understanding of the difficulties and challenges associated with caring for someone with this condition. Or, family involvement may be something much more specific and related to the particular problem area chosen for interpersonal intervention.

In our experience, the education of family members who know little about bipolar disorder when the patient first enters treatment should focus on a number of specific areas. First, it is important to educate family members about what constitutes a major depression, what constitutes an episode of mania, and how one arrives at the diagnosis of bipolar disorder. Second, it is essential that family members and significant others come to understand that no one *chooses* to be depressed and that depressive symptoms are not an attempt to manipulate a family member, to "escape," or to shirk responsibility. However, bipolar patients do sometimes "choose" to be hypomanic. This is easily understandable when one considers the pleasure associated with the hypomanic state, in contrast to the pain of being depressed. It is important, however, for family members to understand that the impaired judgment that is an essential feature of mania and, in some instances, of hypomania, can prevent patients from seeing that their mood or their behavior is out of control. Family members can sometimes play an important role in helping a patient with limited insight to see what is happening. Of course, the efforts of family members to intervene as the patient's mood is escalating can also lead to some of the most severe disputes observed in the families of individuals with bipolar I disorder. Nonetheless, just as a loving family member would attempt to assist someone who has broken a leg in carrying out household tasks that require movement, a loving family member has the same responsibility to *attempt* to assist the individual who is temporarily crippled by lack of insight. The problem, of course, is that the patient with a broken leg is likely to be very appreciative of this assistance, whereas the hypomanic patient is not.

Involvement of family members may also be a more direct part of the interpersonal interventions you undertake with your patient. This is particularly likely to be true when the role disputes problem area is chosen. Indeed, when the focus of treatment is an interpersonal role dispute, it is often extremely helpful to involve the other party to the dispute in one or more of the treatment sessions. This involvement of family members or significant others can simply take the form of trying to understand the dispute from the vantage point of the other party, and thus is just information gathering in nature. Or this involvement may include something more like a brief marital or family therapy intervention, in which you attempt to analyze communication between the parties and suggest strategies for resolving the dispute that both parties to the dispute would be expected to employ in their interactions outside therapy.

SUPPORT GROUPS

Many patients and their family members benefit from participation in support groups. These may be more general support groups for persons with a variety of mental disorders, such as those organized by the United Mental Health Association and the National Alliance for the Mentally Ill (NAMI), or they may be specific to mood disorders or bipolar illness such as those run under the auspices of the Depression and Bipolar Support Alliance (DBSA, formerly the National Depressive and Manic–Depressive Association). These are all national organizations that have hundreds of local affiliates throughout the country. They can usually be located through the telephone directory or via their respective websites. See Appendix 9 for a list of names, addresses, phone numbers, and website addresses for national organizations that sponsor support groups and provide a variety of other support services. In addition, some communities have locally organized support groups that may be run by religious organizations, the YMCA or YWCA, a psychiatric facility, or a community mental health center. Especially for someone participating in an individual therapy like IPSRT, support groups offer the advantage of helping the patient to see that he or she is not alone in suffering with bipolar disorder and that what seem like completely unique and unimaginable experiences have actually been shared by many of those who have the illness. Some patients find the sharing that goes on in a support group enormously relieving; others find the openness and self-disclosure difficult. In deciding whether to recommend that your patient consider joining such a group, you will want to consider how comfortable he or she would be likely to feel in such a situation. Finally, support groups can be a very important adjunct to IPSRT when the interpersonal problem area is one of social isolation (i.e., interpersonal deficit of the isolated type).

Family members may be even greater beneficiaries of what support groups have to offer. Living with a person who has bipolar illness can be a very challenging and frustrating experience. Other family members can be an important source of advice and support in coping with this challenge.

Eventually some patients or family members may take on leadership roles in the support group or in the organizations sponsoring it. Particularly for family members or patients who are now doing well, this can be a very therapeutic experience. The leadership role becomes a source of enhanced self-esteem, and the volunteer activity can help them to feel that something good has come out of having the illness. Now that they are doing well, they can offer something of value to others who are suffering. A caveat: Should your patients become involved in such activity, you will want to monitor the extent to which it leads to overstimulation or to demoralization should they become depressed and unable to carry out the responsibilities of their position. A good way to manage such eventualities is to discuss them ahead of time and to help patients to titrate their volunteer activity to reduce its mania-inducing potential and to anticipate how they will manage or share their responsibilities should they become depressed. The fortunate thing is that in volunteering with mental illness support groups or support organizations, your patient is in an environment where fluctuations in capacities will be well understood by all those with whom he or she is working and supervisors are likely to be glad to spell out contingency plans.

NONSPECIFIC SUPPORT

An essential component of all good management of chronic disease (and bipolar disorder clearly falls into this category) is the provision of nonspecific support. This kind of support is entirely consistent with the therapeutic stance of the IPSRT therapist. It involves displaying a strong interest in the patient and his or her life, especially as affected by the disorder, strong encouragement to stick with treatment even when improvement is not immediate and/or medication side effects are troubling, optimism about the ultimate outcome, and confidence in the patient's ability to make use of the treatment being provided. All of these are implicit in the interpersonal approach on which IPSRT is based. You may find that you will also need to help your patients to navigate the various social services available, including linking them to an intensive case manager or other support services, where appropriate, and encouraging them to make use of services for housing, financing of treatment and other medical care, employment, or education. When the severity of the patient's illness does not warrant such wraparound services, you may still find yourself called upon to help your patient with things such as accessing expensive medications through the indigent programs of various pharmaceutical companies, obtaining medical assistance, and coordinating the patient's physical health care with the care of his or her bipolar disorder. These are activities that many psychotherapists accustomed to working with patients with less severe disorders may not have been called upon to perform; however, unless your patient has an intensive case manager or a physician who has been able to provide this kind of help, these may prove to be key aspects of your care of some patients with bipolar disorder.

Providing IPSRT in any context is likely to prove beneficial to patients with bipolar disorder, but if the goal of treatment is sustained wellness in a patient with a history of multiple recurrences, the contextual elements of treatment are often critical. The more of these elements you (and your collaborating physician, if you have one) can provide, the better your patients' outcomes are likely to be.

The complexity of bipolar illness is such that a wide variety of additional interventions and strategies may be needed to help patients to maintain euthymic mood. We have described some of those that have worked for the patients whom we have treated. If you are an experienced clinician who has treated many patients with bipolar disorder, you undoubtedly have a set of strategies of your own. Some of these will fit well with IPSRT; others may not. If this is a new population for you, then as you become more experienced in working with these patients, you will undoubtedly evolve a set of additional interventions that seem consonant with IPSRT as you do it.

ELEVEN

Monitoring Progress and Enhancing Treatment Adherence

MONITORING SYMPTOMATIC
AND FUNCTIONAL CHANGE IN IPSRT

There is probably no psychiatric disorder in which the regular monitoring of the patient's clinical status is as important as it is in bipolar disorder. In most other disorders, we talk about monitoring "progress," because there is only one direction in which we hope to see symptomatology and functioning move. The challenge in the ongoing assessment of bipolar disorder is that patients can deteriorate in two different directions. Although you want to see the patient who presents in a bipolar depression become less depressed and improve his or her social and occupational functioning, you must always be on guard lest the patient become "too happy" or "too energetic." With the patient who presents in an episode of mania or hypomania, you actually want to see this symptomatology, and even in some cases social and occupational functioning (really overfunctioning), go in the reverse direction. Yet, again, you need to be sure that this quieting of excess enthusiasm and energy doesn't turn into a full-fledged depression.

Furthermore, as a patient stabilizes at something like a euthymic level, you must constantly be monitoring for changes in symptomatology that, again, can go in either direction. Thus, you must constantly keep an eye on both poles of this *bi*polar disorder. You want to facilitate maximal social and occupational functioning, but discourage overfunctioning. You must constantly be on guard for the beginnings of a mania, even in a patient who has not had one for many years.

For these reasons it is essential that, at a minimum, you inquire verbally about the patient's level of depressive and manic/hypomanic symptomatology at each clinical visit.

DISCUSSION OF EARLY WARNING SIGNS
OF IMPENDING EPISODES

You will want to work with your patient, and any available family members or signifi-cant others, to determine exactly how the current episode began, both in terms of early symptoms and in terms of any stressors that might have been related to the onset of the index episode. Was not needing nearly as much sleep as usual the first sign, or was it becoming much more involved in volunteer activities? Did the depression really begin with a change in mood, or did the patient start having trouble with sleep long before any lowering of mood? You should also inquire about the onsets of all previous epi-sodes, if these are not too numerous. If your patient has had multiple previous epi-sodes, inquire about the most recent episodes, being sure to get a sense of how *both* de-pressions and manias begin for this particular patient. You will then work with your patient and available support persons to develop an early response plan: Who in the patient's social network can help the patient recognize the earliest symptoms? What will that person's role be when such symptoms are identified? Where will the patient and/or the family members seek help in the event of the appearance of such symp-toms?

MEASURING SYMPTOMATIC AND
FUNCTIONAL CHANGE IN TREATMENT

Although it is surprising how frequently this is skipped in community practice, from our perspective a careful, systematic review of depressive and hypomanic symptoms at each clinic visit is an essential part of good clinical treatment of any psychiatric disor-der. This review can be done either informally or through a specific rating scale. At a minimum, the review of symptoms should involve asking your patient to rate his or her level of depression and mania or hypomania on a scale of 1–10 for the time period since the last visit. Such symptom review should involve both the symptoms the pa-tient reported at the outset of treatment and other symptoms of depression or mania not reported at that time.

Measuring symptomatic change during treatment can be as simple as asking your patient at each visit to quantify his or her mood on a numerical scale. Depending on your preference and the nature of the patient's recent mood disturbance, you may sim-ply say something like, "With 1 being the most depressed you have ever been and 10 being the best you have ever felt without being high, where would you place your mood in the last week?" If the patient's mood tends to fluctuate frequently, you may prefer to use a scale that goes from –5 (most depressed) to +5 (most manic), with 0 be-ing the sought-after ideal. If the patient is completing SRMs on a regular basis, you can examine the daily mood ratings at the end of the scale and review these during the treatment session. Alternatively, especially if you are interested in targeting change in specific symptoms, you can ask the patient to complete the Beck Depression Inventory (Beck et al., 1961) or the Quick Inventory of Depressive Symptoms (QIDS; Rush et al., 2003), or you can use one of the interview rating scales for depression such as the Ham-ilton Rating Scale for Depression (Hamilton, 1960), the Montgomery–Asberg Depres-sion Rating Scale (Montgomery, 1979), or the Inventory of Depressive Symptoms

(Rush, Carmody, & Reimitz, 2000). Unfortunately, as noted in Chapter 5, there is no comparable self-report scale for mania/hypomania.

Particularly when the frequency of treatment has been reduced to monthly or even more infrequent visits, you may wish to have phone contact with your patient between visits in order to monitor for any symptomatic change. One reason that this kind of contact and monitoring is so essential in this condition is that one of the key features of patients with bipolar disorder is the rapid loss of insight, especially with respect to hypomanic and manic symptomatology. Even the most experienced and well-intentioned patient, the patient who has made a vow never to see the inside of a psychiatric hospital again, almost invariably loses insight about his or her level of symptomatology as mood begins to escalate. This pernicious loss of insight frequently puts you at odds with patients with whom you previously had excellent rapport: He says he has a right to spend a little money now and then; you say, yes, but five new suits in one day seems like more than he can afford (and even if he can afford it, probably represents a symptom of mania/hypomania); she says she has to stay up till 2:00 if she is going to help her kids with their homework and keep the house the way she likes; you say, keeping herself well is more important to her children than cleaning the windows. When this starts to happen, it is an almost certain sign that your patient is already on the road to trouble. By speaking to patients between visits scheduled a month or more apart, you can generally determine within 5 minutes whether all is well or whether it is time to initiate the rescue protocol.

Chapter 5 describes several methods for assessing and monitoring symptoms of depression and mania, as well as methods for monitoring common comorbidities experienced by patients with bipolar disorder. Once you have moved from the initial to the intermediate phase of IPSRT, it may be sufficient simply to review the daily mood ratings that patients complete at the end of the SRM and then to query patients directly during the treatment session, asking them to rate their moods on one of the ordinal scales described in Chapter 5.

Every few sessions, however, it is a good idea to ask patients to complete one of the standardized instruments for depression (the BDI or QIDS) that are described in Chapter 5 in order to obtain information about change in specific symptoms. Because there is no valid and reliable self-report measure of mania/hypomania, at least once every month or two months you will want to conduct one of the clinician-administered assessments for mania/hypomania, such as the Young Mania Rating Scale (Young et al., 1978), to evaluate the presence of individual symptoms of mania and hypomania. As we have often seen, patients can rate themselves as free of manic symptoms on an ordinal scale, while overcharging on their credit cards, becoming involved in foolish business ventures, and getting themselves into all kinds of other trouble. To see whether your patient's mood is becoming more stable over time, you may want to create a chart that looks something like Figure 11.1 (which also appears in Appendix 10 as a blank form for you to copy). The actual numbers you insert on the scale will depend on the specific instrument you use for monitoring depression and mania, but whatever method you chose, this chart can provide you and your patient with a visual representation of progress or change over time.

If you can take the time to calculate your patient's SRM score after each visit, you can make a similar chart for monitoring progress in achieving social rhythm stability. Or you may want to keep the SRM score record on the same chart, as done in Figure

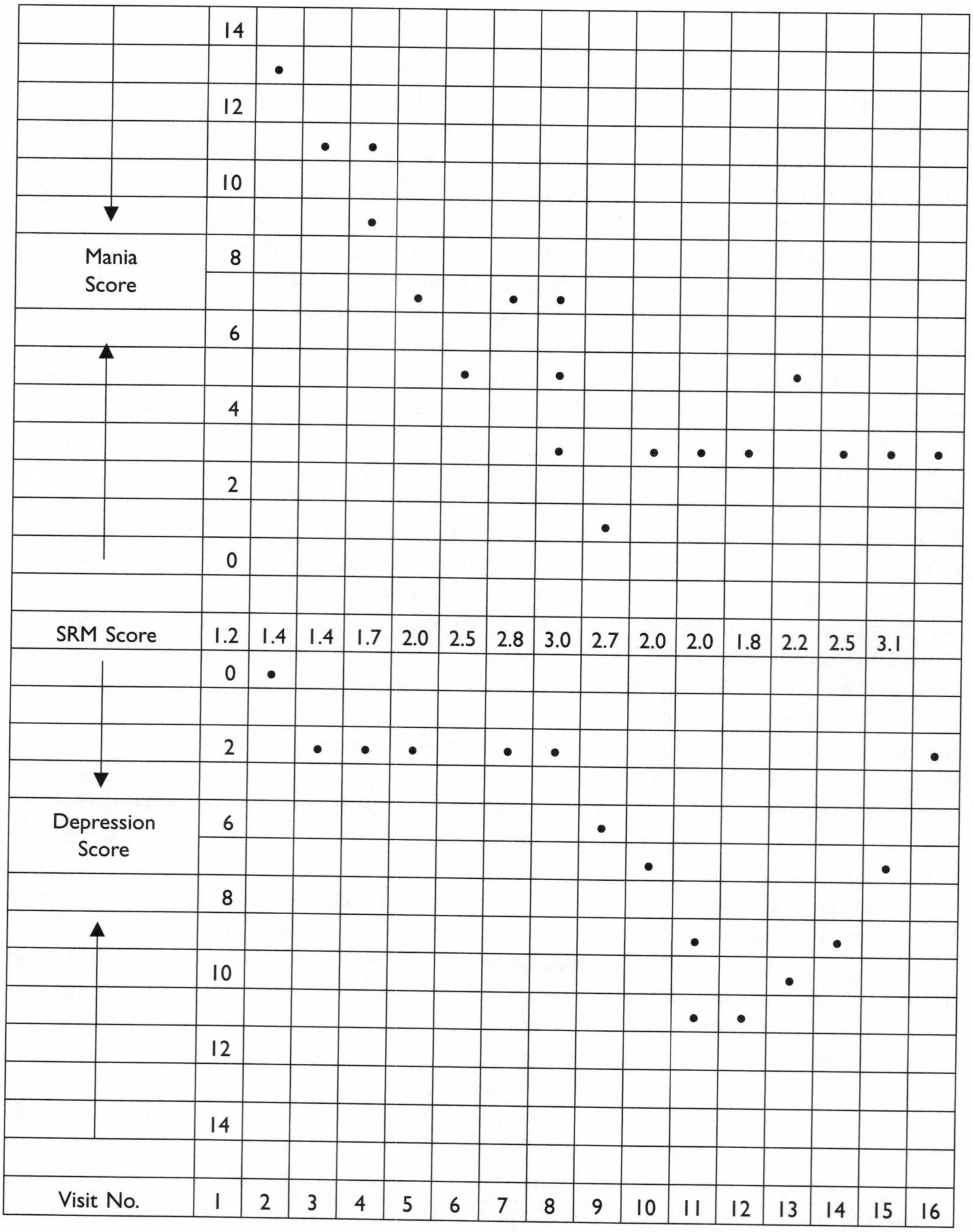

Mania Score (axis labels): 14, 12, 10, 8, 6, 4, 2, 0

SRM Score: 1.2 | 1.4 | 1.4 | 1.7 | 2.0 | 2.5 | 2.8 | 3.0 | 2.7 | 2.0 | 2.0 | 1.8 | 2.2 | 2.5 | 3.1

Depression Score (axis labels): 0, 2, 6, 8, 10, 12, 14

Visit No.	1	2	3	4	5	6	7	8	9	10	11	12	13	14	15	16

FIGURE 11.1. Example of a completed Mood Disorder Monitoring Chart.

11.1. This has the advantage of helping you (and your patient) to see the relationship between changes in rhythm stability and changes in mood. Instructions for calculating the SRM score are provided in Appendices 2 and 4.

Monitoring progress in the area of the patient's social and occupational functioning is likely to be a more highly individualized matter and more closely linked to the interpersonal problem area chosen as the current focus of the interpersonal work. If the interpersonal problem area is *grief*, does the patient seem less sad, and is he more engaged in a social life comparable to that which he enjoyed prior to the loss? Has your patient stopped avoiding people and places that remind him of the deceased? Or, alternatively, has your patient become less involved with rituals (e.g., daily visits to the cemetery, compulsive review of photos or other momentos) that were a feature of his behavior prior to the initiation of the interpersonal work?

If the problem area is *grief for the lost healthy self*, does your patient seem more accepting of her illness and more accepting of the limitations that it places on her? Does your patient, at the same time, seem to understand better the possibilities that do exist for a full and satisfying life despite some limits that the disorder might place on her? Does her adherence to the medication regimen prescribed seem to be improving? How often do you find that the two of you are in conflict about the wisdom of some plan that she has described to you?

Markers of treatment progress can include being able to express sadness about real or presumed losses, becoming more accepting of the fact of having bipolar illness, making life plans that realistically take the illness into account (but do not set unrealistic or unnecessary limits), and working toward those life plans.

When the chosen problem area is *role transitions*, you will want to be monitoring the extent to which the patient seems to have grieved successfully for the lost former role and the extent to which he has engaged in the new role with energy and enthusiasm. Thus, you can ask yourself questions such as the following: Does he continue to dwell on how wonderful life was before he had to conform to the constraints of a full-time job? Does she continue to idealize her life as a nurse, forgetting how incredibly demanding and frustrating that role could be sometimes? Does he still denigrate his new boss and coworkers, or are there some signs of acceptance of his boss's authority and his coworkers' competence? Is she still staying home and watching TV most days, or has she begun to explore some of the volunteer options the two of you have discussed?

The way in which you monitor progress in the role disputes area will depend on the stage of the dispute. If the dispute was active at the time of the initiation of the interpersonal work, you assess progress based on the extent to which the parties to the dispute seem to be getting along better, the extent to which their expectations of one another have become more reciprocal, and the extent to which they are now able to fulfill these more reciprocal expectations. If the dispute is first assessed as being in the impasse phase, initially progress might mean "heating up" the dispute so that the parties are more actively engaged with one another, but not necessarily getting along better. In this phase of the work, you may actually want fairly heated discussion and disagreement between the parties to the dispute. Once they have clearly articulated their expectations of one another, then you can start work on helping them come to some agreement as to which of these expectations they can actually meet and which must be abandoned, at least for the time being. If the relationship is initially assessed to be in the dissolution phase, progress may mean the facilitation of your patient's exit from the relationship. Here your role is to help the patient out of the relationship with the minimum possible psychological distress. If, however, actual exit from the relationship is not possible, as in a parent–child relationship, progress would be marked by acceptance on your patient's part that the relationship is not likely to change, that he or she should reduce or change expectations as to what can be hoped for in the relationship, and move toward other sources of satisfaction. It is worth mentioning here that with patients who have bipolar disorder, you will want to be on the lookout for increases in manic/hypomanic symptoms as well as depression symptoms. Often, the response to such a crisis can paradoxically be a mania rather than a depression.

If *interpersonal deficits* have been chosen as the problem area of focus, progress is likely to be much slower. Typically, patients who present with interpersonal deficits have suffered from these difficulties for many years, if not most of their lives. Therefore, your expectations for change should be modest, even with the type of interpersonal deficit described in the case of Steve in Chapter 9. Even in the case of interpersonal deficits of a more recent nature that are closely linked to a severe episode of mania, we have found that despite the apparent retention of social skills and expressed interest in improved social and occupational functioning, patients of this type may require many, many months of very limited social contact before they feel ready to venture into the social world. One of the clear errors that a novice IPSRT therapist can make is to set expectations too high for the pace at which change can occur in this type of interpersonal deficit work. With patients who have the socially isolated form of deficit, you may base your assessment partially on the patient's increased comfort in interacting with you and partially on the extent to which he or she is socializing outside treatment and how comfortable such experiences are for your patient. With patients who have the chronically unsatisfied or disputatious form of interpersonal deficit, you will base your assessment on the extent to which he or she reports getting along better with family, friends, coworkers, neighbors, and others.

MONITORING AND ENHANCING TREATMENT ADHERENCE

Because patients with bipolar disorder often have a very difficult time with adherence to their pharmacotherapy regimen, improvement in this area is another form of progress you will want to monitor. In fact, there are three aspects of treatment adherence that you will want to attend to in IPSRT treatment of patients with bipolar disorder: medication adherence, completion of the social rhythm metric, and out-of-session work on the selected interpersonal area. With patients suffering from bipolar II disorder, bipolar NOS, or cyclothymia who are not being treated with medication, your attention will need to be focused only on the last two of these areas. We have already described your responsibilities with respect to medication monitoring and setting the stage for adherence to the prescribed medication regimen. To restate the important things that you can do: make certain that your patient agrees with the need for medication and understands the rationale for his or her pharmacotherapy regimen, has some idea (at a layperson's level) of how each medication is expected to work, and is being forthright with you about any uncomfortable side effects that he or she might be experiencing. Patients with bipolar I disorder often require very complex medication regimens, and many patients receive as many as four or five different drugs. Although this kind of polypharmacy is not ideal, it is sometimes necessary to control symptoms. Patients on such complex regimens may need frequent encouragement to stay with their pharmacological treatment. Patients on regimens like this also need frequent evaluation of the kinds of side effects that may occur as a result of *combining* medications. Such side effects are likely to develop slowly, making them harder for the patient to notice. These include gradual, but nonetheless dangerous weight gain, increasingly severe tremor, and actual movement disorders.

As far as out-of-session assignments are concerned, the primary homework assignments in IPSRT are the completion of the Social Rhythm Metric (SRM) and the Likert-type Mood Monitoring Chart. Some IPSRT patients take to the SRM like a "duck to water." These tend to be individuals with a somewhat more compulsive style and those who have felt relatively helpless in the face of their fluctuating mood symptomatology. For such patients, completion of the SRM may represent the first time they have been given an opportunity to do something, other than take medication, to improve the course of their illness. Younger patients, patients who are having difficulty accepting their illness, and particularly those patients who are loath to give up the "spontaneity" of their current lifestyle may well have a very different reaction to the SRM. Such patients need considerable encouragement and therapeutic maneuvering on your part in order to complete the SRM on a regular basis and to make the lifestyle changes that the SRM monitoring implies. As indicated earlier, we have used both a 5-item and a 17-item version of the SRM. The 17-item version has the advantage of giving you a much better sense of the texture of your patient's life. However, completing it on a daily basis represents a considerable commitment on your patient's part.

For those patients who are having difficulty with the SRM, it may be possible to begin with the 5-item version or to switch to it if the patient is failing to complete the 17-item version. With the most dysfunctional patients, we have often limited ourselves to requesting completion of only one or two items, allowing us to concentrate on stabilizing only one or two routines in the first several weeks of treatment. These items have typically been either "good morning time" (the time at which the patient is actually out of bed in the morning) or "good night time" (the time at which the patient puts out the light and attempts to go to sleep). These seem to be the most important routines for stabilizing social rhythms, in part because they tend to determine when so many other social routines (e.g., have breakfast, start work, etc.) are performed, and in part because "good morning time" seems to exert direct effects on the body's circadian system.

If your patient is "resistant" or appears to be having difficulty in completing the SRM, your task is to determine what the reasons for this might be. As implied earlier, the common reasons patients give for failing to complete this homework assignment have to do with denial of the illness in the first place, a general resistance to being in treatment for the illness, and unwillingness to give up the supposed spontaneity of their lives. Depending on which of these problems appears to be most prominent, you might select different strategies and tactics to overcome your patient's difficulty with SRM completion.

If your patient is in general denial of the illness, you might assess the extent to which his or her insight might actually be affected by current symptoms of hypomania. If symptoms do not appear to be interfering, then you might return to the illness history timeline and review with your patient the cost the illness has had in terms of personal growth and development, financial or interpersonal losses, and the like, and review the connection between disruption in social routines and the onset of new episodes. If the problem appears to be more one of unwillingness to give up what your patient perceives as his or her freedom to live more spontaneously than even modest adherence to the general philosophy of social rhythm stabilization would allow, you might use the illness history timeline to try again to help your patient see what the costs of this "free" and "spontaneous" lifestyle have been. You could then go through the kind of decision analysis described in the original IPT Manual (Klerman et al., 1984) to help your patient to determine whether there might be value in giving up some of that "freedom" in exchange for freedom from symptomatology. Above all, you want to be certain that the rationale for the treatment (i.e., how social rhythms affect mood and vice versa) is clear in your patient's mind.

Another strategy that you might try with those patients who are not completing the SRM and mood ratings assignments, is to do what Miklowitz and Goldstein (1997) have referred to as "normalizing the resistance." What they mean by this is to share with your patient your complete understanding of why someone would *not* want to do this relatively tedious task and of how difficult any kind of behavioral change is. You might even share with your patient some difficulty that you have encountered in, for example, making yourself adhere to a healthier diet or exercise more regularly. So, all you really want is for him or her to be direct with you about not being able to do these assignments.

At the same time, you will want to make clear that it has been our experience that those individuals who *do* complete the SRM and mood rating assignments, and who *do* shift to more regular social routines, clearly benefit more from the treatment. In doing so, you might want to use the analogy of the athletic trainer: Individuals who go to a gym on a regular basis are, in general, in better physical condition than those who do not, but those who can afford an athletic trainer (1) are more likely to actually get to the gym on a regular basis and (2) are more likely to complete all of the exercises planned for the day. Your patient can think of completion of the SRM as a kind of free athletic trainer for social rhythm therapy.

In some cases, particularly with older patients who have suffered many episodes of mania and depression and have experienced the cognitive deterioration sometimes associated with long and chronic bipolar illness, SRM completion may simply be too difficult a task. We used to believe that bipolar illness was the "good prognosis" psychotic disorder, in comparison with schizophrenia (which was thought of as the more deteriorative condition); however, we now recognize that a subgroup of individuals with bipolar disorder do experience measurable cognitive deterioration over the years. Patients who have experienced this kind of deterioration may find the completion of the SRM, and particularly the 17-item version, much more than they can manage. With such patients and with patients of limited intelligence, it may be necessary to go to a one- or two-item version of the SRM that queries only about "good morning time" and "good night time." Or it may be preferable simply to make an informal assessment of changes during the treatment session itself. For such patients, you may need to engage a significant other to help them with the task of regularizing their routines. Again, the important thing is to make clear the philosophy of the treatment (in the simplest possible terms) so that your patient understands why he or she is being asked to make these changes.

Yet another possibility to consider when the SRM is not being completed is that the patient is simply too depressed to complete the task. Again, moving from the 17- to the 5-item version or monitoring only one or two symptoms may be of help. Paradoxically, however, for patients who are severely depressed, especially if the depression is of the anergic type, changing social routines, particularly "good morning time" may be one of the most important things you can help your patient to do. Oversleeping, especially oversleeping in the late morning, can have a profoundly depressing effect in patients with mood disorder. Efforts to move your patient's "good morning time" gradually to an earlier and earlier hour are often associated with clear improvement in mood.

CASE EXAMPLE

Johnny was a 41-year-old self-employed carpenter with a 24-year history of untreated bipolar disorder when he entered IPSRT. For most of those 24 years, his close-knit family had simply put up with his "craziness." Sometimes he worked around the clock, finishing more than three normal people could do in twice the time. Other times he would just go to his shop and stare at the TV for hours on end. But somehow he always managed to put food on the table. This time was different, though. Now he wasn't even showering, and it seemed as though he could barely talk. Some days he stayed in bed until 6:00 P.M.. It took two of his brothers to carry him to the car and bring him to the clinic. Johnny's therapist knew that he was barely able to understand what she was saying to him, but it was clear that he understood that he needed help. Rather than even attempting much in the way of assessment or psychoeducation, she decided just to focus first on getting Johnny to establish a regular wake-up time. She enlisted the brothers' help and Johnny's agreement to a plan that involved his getting up each morning at 7:30 and going out for coffee with one or the other of his brothers. She told him that, if at all possible, it would be important for him to try not to go back to bed when he got back home. She told him how hard she knew this would be for him, but that it was his best hope for feeling better quickly. The medications would take at least a few weeks to "kick in." When Johnny and his brothers returned a week later reporting that he had managed to get up and stay up 4 of the last 7 days, she gave him lots of praise. She then asked what had been different about the days on which he could and could not stay up. He was totally confused by this question, but as his therapist did a detailed analysis of what had happened each day after he returned home, Johnny realized that on the days he had managed to stay out of bed, his wife had been in the kitchen when he got home. On the other days, she had been in the basement or at a neighbor's. The therapist then asked Johnny if he thought she could make it a habit to be in the kitchen around the time he was getting back from his coffee "dates." He knew she'd do anything to help. The following week Johnny reported that he had gotten up on time and stayed up for 7 straight days and that his mood was beginning improve just a little. Proceeding at this very slow pace, Johnny's IPSRT therapist continued to work simply on helping him stabilize his wake-up time and then his "good-night time." Within a month, Johnny was well enough that she could return to the other tasks ordinarily associated with the initial phase of IPSRT, such as the completion of the interpersonal inventory and selection of an interpersonal problem area.

A final possibility to consider, particularly in the context of a role dispute or a role transition problem area, is that external circumstances may be preventing the patient from completing the SRM or from being able to adhere to the social rhythm stabilization goals. Engaging your patient in a careful analysis of what interfered on a day-by-day basis with the goals that had been set for social rhythm stabilization may help you to decide on specific ways to intervene interpersonally so that your patient's social routines can become more stable.

ENHANCING ADHERENCE TO WORK ON THE INTERPERSONAL PROBLEM AREA

Although the IPSRT therapist rarely gives specific homework "assignments" relating to the selected interpersonal problem area, the very nature of the treatment, with its emphasis on interpersonal role and relationship change, implies out-of-session activity on the patient's part. This may be in the form of social or occupational activities, or it may be in the form of discussions with significant others. Typically, patients who are doing well in IPSRT return with clear and elaborate descriptions of what they have done between sessions relative to the selected interpersonal problem area.

CASE EXAMPLE

Louise was a 47-year-old homemaker with three grown children. Her younger daughter was still living at home, her older daughter was away at college, and her son had been living on his own for several years, working as a plumber. She had always had a good relationship with her older daughter, but role disputes with her son and younger daughter were the selected problem area during her acute IPSRT treatment. She had done well, from both a symptomatic and an interpersonal perspective, in the acute treatment phase and was now several months into maintenance treatment. She came to her treatment session reporting that she and her younger daughter had driven to visit her older daughter at college. Despite many hours alone in the car together, they had had no major fights and had actually had enjoyed their time alone together. This was a clear change from the past, when they typically could not be alone together for more than a few minutes without fighting. She also reported that she had received her first Mother's Day card ever from her son. She was very pleased by both of these events and told her IPSRT therapist that she thought they represented real progress in her interpersonal therapy goals.

If you find that such progress is not happening, or if your patient repeatedly reports that he or she has been unable to do any of the things that seem to be necessary for change to occur, you might want to consider whether the selected problem area is really the appropriate one for this patient.

After more than 20 years of experience in doing various forms of interpersonal psychotherapy, we have come to recognize that when the treatment is not going well, it is most often because the interpersonal problem area selected is not actually the right one for the particular patient. Sometimes this necessitates an overt discussion with the patient, but sometimes it is simply a matter of reviewing the case in your own mind (or perhaps with a colleague or supervisor) and, without necessarily saying anything directly to your patient, subtly shifting the focus of your work to what you have now concluded is the appropriate problem area.

For example, it is often the case that as you come to know a patient better, you may realize that what appeared at first to be a role disputes case is actually more of an interpersonal deficits case. With further knowledge about your patient's day-to-day life you may see that it is not simply a question of a dispute in one important relationship, but that conflict tends to be a characteristic of almost all of the patient's relationships. In such a case, you would want to continue to focus on helping your patient to resolve the selected dispute, while also pointing out how a lack of reciprocity in role expectations in many of his or her other relationships is leading to conflict.

CASE EXAMPLE

Shawnta was a single 20-year-old African American law student when she entered IPSRT treatment. The interpersonal inventory revealed a highly conflictual relationship with her mother, who was also the caretaker of Shawnta's 4-year-old son. The onset of Shawnta's most recent episode of depression seemed clearly linked to deterioration in this relationship. As Shawnta was dependent on her mother for her son's care and for many other kinds of instrumental support, resolving this role dispute appeared to be critical to her functioning as a law student. After several weeks of IPSRT treatment and long discussions about how she might begin to resolve some of the conflicts she and her mother were having, it became apparent that she was not making any movement in that direction. It also became clear that Shawnta had similar, if less intense, conflicts with many of her professors and fellow students, an aspect that did not emerge in the process of the interpersonal inventory. On further analysis of these conflicts, it became apparent to her therapist that Shawnta had unreasonably high expectations of what others should do for her and little sense that anything, either instrumental or emotional, might be expected of her in return. Having come to this recognition, her therapist shifted the focus of his interventions with Shawnta to one that involved much more in the way of adjusting her expectations from all those around her to be more realistic and helping her to see how having unrealistic expectations of others almost always left her angry and frustrated. At the same time, he shifted his expectation of how quickly change was likely to occur for Shawnta and how much more in-session work would be required on his part to model the behaviors he was hoping Shawnta could learn.

Many things, including the constantly fluctuating symptomatology and the particular temperaments (see Chapter 13) of patients with bipolar disorder, can make the conduct of IPSRT a challenge. Keeping your expectations for treatment adherence reasonable in the context of this illness and returning constantly to the fundamental rationale for the treatment are two strategies that are likely to make IPSRT a more satisfying experience for you and for your patient.

TWELVE

The Therapeutic Relationship in IPSRT

Over the last decade, many different therapists with many different kinds of background and training have conducted IPSRT. To some extent, the nature of their relationships with their patients and the therapeutic stance they have taken have grown out of their specific background and training. It is also the case that different patients will call for different stances in the conduct of this treatment. Finally, the same patient may call for different therapeutic stances, depending on his or her clinical condition at different points in the therapy. Thus, the reality is that there are a variety of general therapeutic stances that seem to work reasonably well in IPSRT, and any given clinician may be called upon to adjust his or her "usual" therapeutic stance as the particular patient or patient's condition warrants.

In general, the therapeutic stance in IPSRT is warm, empathic, and open. However, there are multiple variations in approach. Therapists with backgrounds in social work or nursing probably tend to be more open and self-disclosing, whereas clinicians with psychoanalytic or psychodynamic training may maintain somewhat more therapeutic distance. Above all, the therapeutic stance is one of respect for the patient and admiration for his or her struggle with this challenging illness. In case conceptualization and in the process of treatment, the IPSRT therapist emphasizes the assets (as opposed to the deficits) that the patient brings to the therapy experience and openly supports the patient in his or her efforts at change or maintenance of stability.

The times when you may be called upon to alter your usual therapeutic stance with a patient in IPSRT are typically those involving clinical deterioration. As your patient drifts into depression, you may find that you have to become much more directive than is ordinarily comfortable for you, helping your patient to organize his or her thoughts, to plan a sequence of activities in order to accomplish a goal, and so on. As your patient escalates into hypomania, you may find that you have to be much more confrontative than is typical of your usual therapeutic stance, questioning the wisdom of decisions the patient is making, pointing out the evidence that his or her behavior has changed in ways that could portend disaster. In extreme situations, such as when your patient has clearly become a danger to him- or herself or others or is about to do something that would subsequently prove highly embarrassing, you may even have to be deceptive in order to create a safety net around the patient or to prevent the patient's humiliation.

CASE EXAMPLE

Louisa was a 56-year-old single woman with a 30-year history of severe bipolar disorder. Early in her illness she had had several very protracted hospitalizations, including one lasting over a year. She had alternated between relative euthymia and mild depression for a decade, but had not been hospitalized for more than 12 years. Although she was no longer able to work, she was very well integrated into her neighborhood, with close friends all up and down her street. She took great pride in these relationships and in the fact that many of her friends and neighbors were highly successful professionals who commanded considerable respect in the community. She had been in monthly IPSRT maintenance treatment for several years. She and her therapist had a strong therapeutic relationship based on honesty and mutual respect. When Louisa suddenly became seriously, psychotically manic, her therapist knew that she had to be hospitalized. He also knew that she would never agree to go voluntarily. He had a choice between sending the police to bring her to the hospital and running the risk that she would be humiliated in front of her neighbors, or deceiving her about the need for a lithium blood level (which would necessitate her coming to the clinic even though she had been there only the week before) and running the risk of a serious rupture in their relationship. He chose the latter course, making certain that the police would be ready to escort her from the outpatient clinic to the hospital should she (as he suspected she would) refuse to go. In the end, she agreed to be escorted to the hospital by the police rather than be taken involuntarily, but was absolutely furious at her therapist and remained so for much of her inpatient stay. Only when she returned home and had a chance to think about what it would have been like to have the police come for her at her house was she able to express her gratitude to her therapist for his thoughtful and considerate deception.

What can make maintaining one particular therapeutic stance difficult with patients suffering from bipolar disorder, whether it be in the context of IPSRT or some other treatment, is the extraordinary variability in clinical presentation even within the same patient. Perhaps the word that best characterizes the ideal therapeutic stance in IPSRT is "flexible." One week your patient may be irritable, but trusting. A week later that same patient can be irritable and highly suspicious of you. The first week, you may be able to confront your patient about his irritability and ask how it is interfering in his life, what would help to reduce it, and how you could be helpful in the process. At the next visit, this same approach might be a disaster, as your motives for wanting to help at all become a source of contention.

The temporal focus in IPT and in IPSRT remains consistently on the present and the future. It is perhaps this insistent focus on present difficulties and future goals that is one of the secrets of the success of the interpersonal therapies. This is not to say that no reference is ever made to the past or that the IPSRT therapist *ignores* information about past clinical history or past relationships. Much to the contrary, it has always been our contention that the best IPT and IPSRT therapists keep past history very much in mind as they are helping the patient to ameliorate problems in the present and prevent problems in the future. However, once the initial phase of treatment has been completed, overt allusions to past interpersonal experiences are generally kept to a minimum, except as they might be needed occasionally to help your patient understand why he or she is behaving in a paradoxical way in the present. Even then, the IPSRT therapist tries to keep the therapeutic focus on the present while formulating hypotheses as to why the patient is behaving in a paradoxical fashion, based on an understanding of his or her past interpersonal history. It is our suspicion that an intensive focus on the past, particularly on problems and unpleasantness in the past, can only serve to increase rumination and depressive affect. Thus, we try hard to remain present-focused and positive about the patient's ability to make the kinds of changes we have agreed will lead to improved mood and interpersonal satisfaction. In some respects, you might think of yourself as a cheerleader in a fairly literal sense for your patient. Like the cheerleaders at a football game who are focused on the players, you are focused on the patient's potential and what he or she can do in the subsequent moments, days, and weeks to improve his or her "score."

CASE EXAMPLE

Defne was a 29-year-old married woman of Turkish origin who presented for IPSRT treatment accompanied by her bewildered husband. They had immigrated to the United States approximately 1 year before. She had recently experienced her first manic episode, which lasted only a few weeks, and then cycled into a severe depression. Previously, she had made a good adaptation to her new surroundings. Although her English was limited when she first arrived in the United States, she had learned it quickly. She soon was able to shop on her own and to cook from American recipes, deal with English-speaking repairmen, and generally manage on her own. She found work as a data entry clerk, but remained socially isolated even though there were a number of other young women in similar circumstances in the apartment building where she and her husband lived.

Her early history was one of trauma and abuse. She was the youngest of seven girls, all of whom were severely mistreated by a father who had wanted only sons and had none. Her mother had been depressed for as long as Defne could remember and had been unable to protect her daughters from the father's verbal and physical abuse. At the outset of treatment she was spending much of her unstructured time ruminating about these childhood experiences, and this was what she wanted to talk about in therapy. Her IPSRT therapist correctly assessed that a focus on these experiences was unlikely to be beneficial for Defne. Even though Defne had initially made a superficially good transition to life in the United States, her therapist conceptualized the interpersonal problem area as an incomplete role transition. She spent several sessions pointing out in minute detail how much Defne had accomplished since coming to this country: She had found an apartment, negotiated the lease, gotten a phone installed, learned where to buy all the things she needed, adapted her homemaking to American products and appliances and even gotten a good job with a decent benefit package, something many young American women have difficulty doing. The therapist's only reference to Defne's past was her discussion of how much strength and support Defne had drawn from her sisters during her childhood and in the first years of her marriage. She helped Defne to see that even though she had a very good marriage, she also needed female companionship. As Defne's depression began to lift, the therapist encouraged her to reach out to some of the women in her apartment building. At each step along the way, she kept the focus on Defne's remarkable strengths and provided ample amounts of praise for each small accomplishment.

In IPSRT, there is rarely an overt focus on the therapeutic relationship unless the interpersonal problem area is interpersonal deficits. Nonetheless, the therapist's open, supportive stance and the reciprocal nature of the exchange between the therapist and the patient can and should mirror the quality of the relationships your patient is seeking outside therapy. As you set reasonable expectations for what the patient should be doing in the therapy and the patient is able to fulfill them, as you clarify the patient's expectations of you and as the patient sees that you are fulfilling these expectations for help with his or her bipolar disorder, you are modeling the kind of relationship characterized by reciprocity of expectations that is the interpersonal psychotherapy ideal. In the original 1984 manual, Klerman and colleagues state that role disputes arise from "non-reciprocal role expectations." There is a world of wisdom packed into that three-word phrase. In other words, in any relationship, things go well when each party has a clear idea of what his or her role in the relationship should be and what the role of the other person should be, and each is able to meet the other's expectations without having to give up his or her own. Things go badly when the parties don't have the same role expectations and/or when one or both parties cannot meet the expectations of the other. This can certainly be true of therapeutic relationships and is likely to lead dissatisfaction and, eventually, to dropout. Unfortunately, many aspects of the specific psychopathology of bipolar disorder and the complexity of its treatment can interfere with the development of the ideal, reciprocal-expectations-met therapeutic relationship.

PROBLEMS IN THE THERAPEUTIC RELATIONSHIP

Clearly, the instability of mood that characterizes bipolar disorder can lead to substantial problems in the therapeutic relationship. A consistent feature of that mood instability, whether the patient be manic, hypomanic, or depressed, is irritability. Thus, if your patient is struggling with either pole of the illness, he or she may find it very difficult, if not impossible, to control feelings of irritability. This can lead to overtly nasty behavior toward you, toward support staff, or toward others in the clinic or waiting room and can make for very difficult clinical interactions. If a patient appears particularly irritable on a given day, you may elect to point this out directly or you may simply elect to be somewhat less challenging and demanding in that particular session. What is frequently quite helpful is to try to help the patient understand what the particular source of the irritability is, if one exists.

CASE EXAMPLE

Regina, a 61-year-old woman whose bipolar disorder had been in remission for several years, came to her IPSRT session complaining overtly of irritability. She was well aware that she was giving everyone, including her therapist and the clinic staff, a terrifically hard time. She was particularly distressed by the fact that she was irritable with an old friend of her mother's who was in the hospital being treated for a brain cancer. This woman was the last of her mother's circle of friends who remained alive and had been a great support to Regina after her mother had died. Now, however, this woman was seemingly unappreciative of Regina's phone calls and visits, while nonetheless making clear demands that Regina call and visit her on a regular basis. Regina's therapist asked a number of questions about this woman, her relationship to Regina, and her current medical condition. It soon became clear that much of Regina's irritability grew out of her fear and anger that this woman was going to die. Once she understood what it was that she was really upset about, and once she was able to concede that her mother's friend was probably not able to show more enthusiasm or appreciation, Regina found she was better able to control her irritability both with her mother's friend and with her therapist.

If there doesn't appear to be any identifiable source of the irritablility, simply reminding your patient that this is a waxing and waning feature of the illness that can be expected to subside eventually can be a helpful intervention. As implied earlier, this approach can work well if your patient is not simultaneously paranoid, but will require a different set of tactics if he or she is particularly suspicious.

Certain temperamental features that seem to characterize a substantial proportion of patients with bipolar disorder can also make the therapeutic relationship quite challenging. Perhaps because many patients with bipolar disorder have had psychotic experiences that others have never had, or perhaps because many patients with bipolar disorder have had either the great personal or familial success that often accompanies the energy and enthusiasms of bipolar disorder, a subset of patients with bipolar I disorder present with an entitled stance that is rarely seen in other outpatient populations. This may mean that unlike your less demanding, even self-effacing, patients with unipolar disorder or panic disorder, your IPSRT patients will sometimes expect that you remember every detail of their histories, that you are never late for an appointment, that you never cancel or change an appointment, and so on. When such patients are completely euthymic (and not irritable), it may be possible to make this a therapeutic issue; however, when patients evidence this kind of entitled behavior, sometimes there is nothing that can be done other than to apologize for this "affront." If the moment seems right, however, it may be very helpful to your patient to discuss your reactions to his or her feelings of entitlement and to inquire whether this kind of behavior may be having an impact on relations with friends, family members, colleagues, or even important service people like the patient's regular bus driver or mailman. Obviously, such a discussion must be approached with great care, but when it goes well, it can actually lead to real improvement in the patient's quality of life because others become more willing to engage in those desired reciprocal relations with the patient. The good news is that this stance typically waxes and wanes with changes in mood symptomatology and is unlikely to represent an ongoing threat to the therapeutic relationship.

An elaboration and extension of this entitled stance can sometimes be a high degree of litigiousness on the part of some patients with bipolar disorder. A forewarning that this might be the case is information gathered in the course of completing the illness history timeline, indicating that the patient has been involved in multiple lawsuits, public complaints, letter writing campaigns, and the like. If this proves to be the case, you might want to consider whether you want to take this patient on in the first place, as it is not unlikely that you will become the focus of such a lawsuit or become embroiled in a lawsuit that the patient is currently pursuing or planning against someone else. This is not to say that the courts are not an appropriate venue for righting some of the many wrongs done to individuals who have bipolar disorder; however, you should use your best clinical judgment as to how likely it is that a particular patient will attempt to involve you in matters in which you do not wish to become involved. Thus, when you have a suspicion that litigiousness may be an issue, you will want to be especially specific in your discussions with such a patient about the nature of your record keeping and what his or her rights are with respect to access to your or your agency's or hospital's records. Be particularly careful in your documentation of this conversation and in your documentation of the treatment in general.

Issues relating to confidentiality can become a problem in the therapeutic relationship with virtually any patient with bipolar disorder. Manic–depressive illness is a much more stigmatized condition than many of the disorders we deal with on an outpatient basis. Patients with bipolar disorder are well aware of this stigma; thus, they may be much more sensitive than many of your other patients to having it known that they are in treatment, to being acknowledged by a therapist should they be encountered in public, and so forth. For this reason you will want to be particularly clear with patients in IPSRT about what your specific policies are with respect to confidentiality, especially as it involves family members, friends, and employers. At the University of Pittsburgh, where IPSRT was developed, we have taken a very strong stand that, like other chronic diseases, bipolar disorder is best managed in an atmosphere that keeps family members, friends, and sometimes even employers closely involved and cognizant of what is going on in the treatment. We have taken the position that once the patient has given us permission to communicate with a family member or friend, nothing about the treatment will be kept confidential except what the patient specifically asks us to keep confidential. We feel that this policy leads to the best patient care and the most successful management of recurrent mood disorders. However, there are patients who may find this management method inconsistent with their feelings and desires. All this should be clarified as early in the treatment relationship as possible. As mentioned earlier, you will also want to establish early in treatment how your patient would prefer you to handle any chance encounters while out in public. Often patients with bipolar disorder will be fine with the idea of being greeted if they are alone, but would prefer that you not acknowledge them if they are with others.

The management of suicidal thinking and suicidal behavior is another substantial challenge for the therapeutic relationship with patients with bipolar disorders. Individuals who suffer from bipolar I and bipolar II disorders are at the highest risk of all psychiatric patients for completed suicide, meaning that the management of suicide in this population takes on a very particular level of significance. You will *absolutely* want to establish a level of openness between you and your patient with respect to suicidal thinking and plans. If a patient doesn't feel comfortable being open with you about these issues, it will clearly be impossible to do an adequate job of protecting that patient. Yet your overreacting to suicidal thinking may lead to your patient to shutting down and not being open with you about this in the future. This possibility, then, must be handled with a great deal of delicacy and thoughtfulness. If you are not the patient's pharmacotherapist, you will want to have a clear agreement with whoever is managing the patient's medications as to how you will jointly respond to suicidal thinking. You must also be clear in your own mind about your level of willingness to breach your patient's confidentiality to protect him or her against suicide, and you will probably want to be explicit with your patients about what your policy is in this regard at a time when they are *not* suicidal. Reviewing this issue when patients *are* expressing suicidal thinking, however, can have the unintended effect of preventing you from effectively protecting them, because they then refuse to be honest with you about these feelings. Finally, as indicated earlier, unless you are providing the patient's pharmacotherapy yourself, you will need a good relationship with your patient's pharmacotherapist. Under the best of circumstances, you would be in regular communication with your patient's pharmacotherapist and have easy and immediate access to him or her if your patient's clinical condition changes. Should you find yourself taking on a patient whose physician is reluctant to establish this kind of open communication or seems uninterested in your view of how your patient is doing, you may want to consider whether you can provide a safe treatment context for that patient. As mentioned earlier, IPSRT provided in any context is probably better than no IPSRT at all; however, poor communication or the absence of communication with your patient's physician certainly represents a less than ideal context for IPSRT.

If you plan on seeing multiple patients with bipolar disorder, you may consider creating a personal referral list of several physicians who seem skilled in working with patients with bipolar disorder and who are collaborative in their approach. If a patient comes to you without a prescribing physician or indicates that he or she is considering changing physicians, you can then refer your patient to one of these colleagues. If patients with bipolar disorder become a large part of your practice, you may find that limiting your referrals for pharmacotherapy to one or two colleagues, with whom you can have regular contact to discuss your shared cases and general management strategies is the ideal situation. Under these circumstances, you should be able to get a good sense of what your colleague is likely to do in any given clinical situation and be able to anticipate for your patient the probable next steps. Likewise, your colleague is likely to be able to anticipate how you would wish to handle most problems that come up and is, therefore, able to set the stage for your interventions.

THIRTEEN

Poor Outcome and How to Handle It

Data on the clinical epidemiology of bipolar disorder make it clear that even under ideal treatment circumstances (i.e., guideline pharmacotherapy and manual-driven, empirically supported psychotherapy), outcomes for a subset of patients with bipolar I disorder remain poor. Given our current therapeutic armamentarium, there seem to be limits on the extent to which any intervention or set of interventions can lead to sustained periods of euthymia in some patients with bipolar disorder. In many cases, however, patients who appear difficult to treat may experience clear benefit from modifications of their treatment regimen.

As one must do with all "treatment-resistant" patients, the IPSRT therapist's first job is to evaluate the potential source(s) of difficulty. Has the patient been properly diagnosed? Is the patient experiencing either iatrogenic or organic medical problems? Is there a comorbid alcohol or substance abuse problem that complicates treatment or treatment adherence? Are there psychotherapeutic issues that should be addressed in a new or different manner? Have you inadvertently chosen the wrong IPSRT problem area? Was the problem area the correct one for the initial focus of treatment, but is no longer appropriate? Is an occult comorbid condition emerging as the initial condition comes under better control? Is that comorbid condition one that you are not fully trained to treat?

Because patients with bipolar disorder are diagnostically complicated, at high risk for medical comorbidities, and usually on complex pharmacotherapeutic regimens, the process of determining sources of treatment difficulty requires careful collaboration with the treating physician if you yourself are not providing the pharmacotherapy. The nonphysician clinician's role when treatment response is less than ideal is a very important one, because the therapist typically spends more time with the patient than does the pharmacotherapist and is often the first member of the treatment team to recognize deterioration or failure to improve. Moreover, because of the therapist's generally greater familiarity with the patient's day-to-day life, he or she is likely to have more hypotheses about what the sources of the difficulty might be and is in a better position to explore when no such hypotheses come readily to mind.

MISSING THE LONG-TERM PERSPECTIVE

Because as IPSRT therapists we focus intensely on the patient's present and future life, there is a risk of missing clues that come from the patient's past. Even though we may see patients over many months or years, we have only a cross-sectional view of our patients' lives.

CASE EXAMPLE

When she began IPSRT treatment, Carolyn was an obese 47-year-old woman with bipolar I disorder and a history of alcohol abuse. She was being treated with sodium divalproex and IPSRT. Carolyn had worked intermittently as a paralegal for a law firm that had its offices near her home. At the time she entered treatment, she was on medical leave because of a debilitating episode of depression. Carolyn had mentioned early in her treatment that since achieving sobriety a decade earlier, she had gained more than 100 pounds, but her therapist really could not envision what she might have looked like before she stopped drinking.

While Carolyn was on sodium divalproex, her weight continued to rise, despite her efforts to diet. She and her therapist agreed to focus on a role transition in the domain of work: She began to recognize that the demands of being a paralegal were unmanageable with her bipolar disorder and that she needed to seek a less stressful job. Although Carolyn initially made slow but steady improvement in other areas of her life after starting IPSRT, her job-hunting efforts were surprisingly feeble. Initially it wasn't clear why Carolyn seemed to be avoiding the few job interviews she got and appeared to be unable to push her resume more aggressively, despite her precarious financial situation. It was only when her therapist tried to walk her step-by-step through the process of getting ready for and going to a job interview that he became aware of what was really standing in her way. Through that process, it became clear to both Carolyn and her therapist that where she was stuck was in getting dressed for these interviews. She still remembered that 135-pound young woman who first presented herself for a job at the law firm where she had worked and how she had felt about herself going for that interview. Her current weight contributed to tremendous shame about her body and made her reluctant to expose herself to the perceived humiliation of interviewing with a new employer. It was one thing at the law firm: The people there seemed not to notice how overweight she had become, or they were too polite to say anything. But the idea of having to put herself together to interview with new people was something she could hardly bring herself to think about. Once this was all clear, Carolyn's therapist encouraged her to relay her concerns about her weight to her physician. He responded by adding topiramate to her medication regimen, checking her thyroid function tests (which turned out to be borderline abnormal) and referring the patient to a weight management program. He told her that he would continue to monitor her thyroid function and would consider supplementation if her values did not normalize. As Carolyn began to lose weight, she felt more comfortable in pursuing job options and more optimistic that she could get the help and support of her treatment team in improving her appearance.

CHANGES IN DRUG METABOLISM

Although some problems in therapy or in the course of your patient's bipolar illness can be handled well by a shift in the focus of the interpersonal work, sometimes what is required is a change in pharmacotherapy or other somatic interventions. Even though you may not be the prescribing physician, often you will be seeing your patients more frequently and for considerably longer sessions than their pharmacotherapists. This puts you in an excellent position to observe subtle changes in your patients' moods and to offer suggestions for changes in their pharmacotherapy.

CASE EXAMPLE

Lydia is a 67-year-old patient with a 40-year history of bipolar I disorder who is unable to take lithium or any of the other so-called mood stabilizers. As a result, she has been treated for many years with a combination of neuroleptic and the tricyclic antidepressant, nortriptyline. Despite an early history characterized by multiple severe depressions and several suicide attempts, this treatment combination had enabled her to maintain a relatively euthymic mood for many, many years. One of the positive features of nortriptyline as an antidepressant is that it has a very specific therapeutic window in which serum levels should fall for the treatment to be maximally effective. After many months of stability, Lydia appeared for her regular visit with her IPSRT therapist complaining of everything but depression: She had had a bad argument with a neighbor with whom she usually got along well, she had been unable to find anything she was looking for at the grocery store, she had a million errands to run but couldn't motivate herself to get even one of them completed, and so forth. Despite the fact that Lydia denied any clear change in her mood, Lydia's IPSRT therapist correctly assessed that her patient was more depressed and irritable than was typical. Her therapist suspected that her antidepressant level had dipped below the therapeutic window and suggested this possibility to Lydia. At first, Lydia dismissed the possibility, pointing to all her "justifiable reasons" for being in such a bad mood. When the therapist then pointed out that she had handled similar and much worse frustrations in the past without becoming angry or irritable, Lydia was forced to admit that maybe he had a point. At least she was willing to entertain the possibility.

Because her therapist worked in a hospital setting, he knew that it would be possible to have blood drawn for a serum nortriptyline level that day. He put in a call to Lydia's pharmacotherapist, with whom he collaborated closely, and she agreed that it made sense to evaluate their patient's blood level. Within 48 hours, the results had come back. Although there had been no change in Lydia's diet, no increase in her smoking, and no change in other factors that might affect her blood level, indeed Lydia's serum nortriptyline level was now clearly below the lower limit of the therapeutic window. Her pharmacotherapist immediately ordered an increase in her dose. Within a matter of days, Lydia was beginning to feel better.

What Lydia's case also illustrates is the value of close collaboration between psychotherapist and pharmacotherapist in the treatment of bipolar disorder. Had that relationship not been one of mutual respect in which the psychotherapist felt confident to make a recommendation to the physician and she, in turn, felt confident of the therapist's assessment, the outcome might have been very different for Lydia. What turned out to be only a minor "blip" could instead have deteriorated into a protracted episode of depression had this level kind of collaboration not existed. When such collaboration is not possible, IPSRT therapists can help to teach patients how to be their own advocates with their doctors regarding preventative medication changes and other aspects of their pharmacotherapy. Indeed, teaching patients to establish this kind of relationship with their pharmacotherapists is a good idea even when the IPSRT therapist and pharmacotherapist collaborate frequently and effectively. When the pharmacotherapist is unwilling to collaborate either with the therapist or with the patient in this way, the therapist's role may be to help the patient make a transition to another physician if that is possible under the terms of the patient's health care coverage.

SEASONAL MOOD VARIATION

Bipolar disorder is cyclical in nature, and patients and therapists often struggle to understand the poor outcomes of treatment. Is there a pattern to the changes, or are they completely random? Many patients with bipolar disorder have a seasonal pattern to their illness. In these cases, changes in medication, psychotherapy foci and, especially, SRM work may need to vary, depending on the season of the year. Therapy can fail if therapists do not get an accurate history of the patient's prior illness course that takes into account seasons of the year (something to look for when completing the illness history timeline at the outset of treatment) and do not apply that information in their work with their patients.

CASE EXAMPLE

Janis was a 40-year-old single woman with bipolar I disorder when she began treatment with IPSRT. She entered treatment in early December in an episode of depression that had been ongoing for several months. She reported a history of bipolar disorder beginning in her early 20s, with yearly episodes of both mania and depression that clearly had a seasonal pattern. Her mood began to dip each September, with worsening symptoms over the fall. Her mood tended to lift in mid-February, and by April she experienced hypomanic symptoms. She first sought treatment for her bipolar disorder when she was 35, but had not seen much real improvement since starting pharmacotherapy.

At first, all went well with her IPSRT treatment. Janis was desperate to get some relief from her depression. She worked hard on the behavioral activation aspects of IPSRT, and her blood levels suggested that she was taking her medication regularly. By Christmas, she was feeling much better, and by the end of January she reported essentially euthymic mood. She was energetically engaged in efforts directed toward a role transition from an unsatisfying job that she and her therapist had identified as the most important focus of her therapy. It was a real pleasure to work with her. Within 2 months, however, she was irritable, unreasonable, and turning off the very people whose help she needed to effect this role transition. When her IPSRT therapist did a systematic evaluation of her mood symptoms using the Young Mania Rating Scale, Janis scored an 18, well into the seriously hypomanic range. Her therapist knew from her illness history timeline that this had been her manic time of year, but that was before she began taking medication. Although, up to this point, Janis had been a model patient, her therapist wondered whether she was continuing to adhere to her pharmacotherapy. When he confronted her about the possibility that this might not just be a season-of-the-year effect, Janis acknowledged that since first going on medications she had always discontinued them on her own in the early spring because she missed the hypomanic surge she had always had at that time of year. She admitted that her hypomanic mood state was addicting.

Her IPSRT therapist retrieved the illness history timeline they had completed when they first began therapy and noted these instances of medication discontinuation. He also pointed out that her worst manias had actually occurred in association with medication discontinuation, manias that had cost her good jobs and good friendships. He asked Janis to describe in detail a typical period of hypomania. It turned out that although most of these periods had been associated with much productivity and energy, they had also been associated with a lot of conflict both at work and in her personal life. He asked if she thought those few weeks of hypomania were worth the price she had often paid for them. This work enabled the patient to gain insight into the real consequences of her noncompliance and the consequences of her manias and hypomanias. It also enabled Janis to give up idealizing the hypomanias.

In addition to insisting that she contact her physician and restart her medication, Janis's therapist then worked with her to anticipate her mood cycles. Exploring the early warning signs of the hypomanias and catching the mood change early was key to helping Janis achieve more stability. Once Janis restarted her medication, they watched for early warning signs and were able to discuss this with her treating psychiatrist, who made some medication adjustments. Her therapist stressed the importance of stabilizing her sleep–wake schedule and the importance of not fooling herself into thinking she did not need her sleep, especially in her vulnerable time of year. In addition, he worked with the SRM and with schedule planning in general to encourage her not to plan major trips during this period and to avoid engaging in extra activities that might be particularly stimulating. He worked with her to identify relaxing, self-soothing activities and to pace herself when she needed or wanted to be involved in something more stimulating. Her illness history timeline indicated that Janis had often begun a romantic relationship during this vulnerable period. Such relationships were intense and developed too quickly. Her therapist discussed how this pattern was both a result of her mood elevation and a contributor to it. He cautioned her about getting overinvolved in new relationships in early spring. Janis was able to use the therapy to evaluate this pattern and slow down the pace of new relationships.

A few months later, Janis and her therapist also evaluated the seasonal pattern of her depressions, which began in early fall. The therapist used the SRM to help Janis with behavioral activation as fall approached, again regulating her sleep–wake cycle, but here pointing out the need to motivate herself to keep her schedule stable. Janis decided to enroll in an exercise class that met twice a week to help prevent her from isolating herself and to keep her energy more constant. They worked in advance of the fall to help her organize her schedule so that she would not overwhelm herself with activities or responsibilities that she would not be able to complete. As with her hypomania symptoms, the therapist worked with Janis to understand the early warning symptoms of depression and encouraged her to discuss them with her psychiatrist. In October, Janis experienced what looked like the beginning of a depressive episode. An antidepressant medication was added to her treatment regimen. She was able to follow the schedule previously outlined, and she experienced a much less intense and much briefer "depression" than that of the prior year. The fact that she had not suffered through several months of severe depression that winter also made her less desperate for her hypomania once spring arrived. The following July, Janis could look back on the first year of real stability she had had in her adult life.

WHEN SYMPTOMS ARE BEYOND THE CONTROL
OF OUTPATIENT TREATMENT

Even with the most dedicated treatment team, patients can experience severe exacerbations of their bipolar illness that are beyond the reach of either medication or psychotherapy. When this occurs, sometimes hospitalization is necessary. In many cases, patients will concur with the need for more intensive treatment and even be relieved by the suggestion of hospitalization; however, in other cases you may be called upon to initiate an involuntary hospitalization. This can be a very frightening and threatening experience for a therapist, particularly when the therapeutic relationship is a long-standing one and there has been a high degree of trust between the therapist and the patient. There are times when this may involve bringing the patient to the therapy session under what one might call false pretenses, with the therapist knowing that an order for involuntary hospitalization has already been obtained and that police will be at the clinic or the therapy office to transport the patient to a hospital. At other times, it may involve sending the police to a patient's home in order to transport him or her to the hospital. These are always very difficult decisions to make. They can sometimes be made easier if the therapist is working in collaboration with a physician and the physician concurs with the need for involuntary hospitalization. They can also be made easier if the therapist has the concurrence of family or friends that hospitalization is necessary.

What can make this kind of intervention especially difficult is that, because of the high levels of irritability associated with bipolar disorder, the amount of hostility and anger directed at those initiating the involuntary hospitalization can be truly monumental. In our experience, when therapists are able to persist in the face of that kind of anger and hostility, are able to visit the patient regularly in the hospital, and can see the patient through to an appropriate discharge, in the end patients are grateful for having been cared for in this way.

CASE EXAMPLE

Angelo was a 20-year-old male attending a local technical school who was brought to see his former therapist by his very concerned parents. Angelo had stopped going to classes, was talking incessantly about women whom he had met at a night club, and was sleeping very little. Although he had been treated for depression for several years while in high school, he had never experienced symptoms of mania or hypomania. It was clear to the therapist that Angelo was manic. She attempted to convince him that he needed to be seen by a psychiatrist, that he needed medication. Even though Angelo had always liked and trusted his former therapist, he was having none of this. He had very little insight into his condition and was quite grandiose. He refused to see a psychiatrist, insisting, "Nothing is wrong with me. This is the best I've ever been!" The therapist and his parents were very worried about Angelo, but there was no evidence of the kind of dangerous behavior that would allow the therapist to initiate an involuntary hospitalization.

The therapist agreed to stay in close contact with the parents, who made an appointment with a psychiatrist despite their son's protestations. The next day, Angelo's condition had deteriorated even further. He had not slept at all the night before, was convinced that he was destined to save all of his grade school friends from their troubles with the law and with the opposing neighborhood gang, and was drawing designs for a large tattoo he planned to have applied to his face. What was most worrying was that his temper was becoming more and more explosive. Still, there were no clear grounds for hospitalization, and Angelo was more convinced than ever that nothing was wrong with him. The following day the therapist received a phone call from Angelo's parents reporting that they had found several guns in the back of their car after their son had gone out for the evening with "friends." Angelo insisted that he was keeping the guns to help out his friends. The therapist felt that this was evidence of potentially life-threatening poor judgment. Knowing that it might jeopardize her formerly good relationship with Angelo, she nonetheless agreed to meet Angelo and his frightened parents at a local emergency room to initiate an involuntary admission.

WHEN FEELINGS ABOUT THE PATIENT
INTERFERE WITH TREATMENT

Another potential source of poor outcome in IPSRT are the therapist's feelings about the patient, or what is referred to as therapist countertransference—either negative or positive. For instance, a therapist may feel especially hopeless about a patient who has had a long and difficult course of illness and fail to recognize and build upon the patient's remaining strengths. Alternately, the therapist's feelings for or identification with a likable patient—perhaps someone with whom the therapist shares a professional background or personal characteristics—may cause him or her to set unrealistically high goals for the patient. As in any psychotherapy, the therapist is responsible for identifying his or her own feelings about a patient and ensuring that those feelings do not interfere with the patient's treatment. Additional supervision—even for the experienced therapist—can be quite helpful in identifying countertransference as a source of a therapeutic impasse.

CASE EXAMPLE

Jayna was a 21-year-old woman with a history of bipolar disorder who had her first episode of illness at 13. Having lost years of critical development to her illness, she acted much younger than her 21 years and was extremely dependent on her overwhelmed single mother. Her mother prepared all her meals, roused her in the morning, and essentially expected nothing of her daughter. Jayna was ambivalent about her dependence on her mother. On one hand, she wanted to act like a "grownup"; on the other hand, she seemed unable to take any responsibility for herself. After months of talking about these issues with Jayna in the context of helping her resolve the role dispute with her mother, her therapist began to feel demoralized. Although each week Jayna said in session that she would help around the apartment, look for work, set her own alarm clock, and so forth, she never did any of these things. Her therapist began to feel angry at Jayna for her inability to make any changes. The therapist appropriately identified these feelings in herself and did her best to prevent her own feelings from entering the treatment, trying each week to break the tasks down into smaller and more manageable components. This went on for many months with no observable change in Jayna's behavior.

Just when it appeared that Jayna might finally be making some progress, however, she came to her session and announced quite unexpectedly that she was going to marry a neighborhood boy who was joining the military—someone her therapist had never even heard about! Jayna's plan was to relocate with him to another state soon after the wedding. Although her therapist believed that this was not a healthy move for Jayna, she did little to intervene actively with the patient's plans. Within a few months Jayna was married and had left treatment. In retrospect, the therapist wondered if her frustration with Jayna and her resulting negative feelings about her prevented her from helping Jayna to truly understand the risks she was taking by marrying a relative stranger and expecting him to care for her as her mother had done.

What Jayna's case also illustrates is how therapy can go awry when the wrong problem area is selected. The interpersonal problem area chosen by Jayna's therapist (and agreed upon by Jayna) was role disputes with her mother. At an intellectual level, Jayna could agree that her mother's expectations of her, a 21-year-old, were perfectly reasonable, but she was still unable to implement the changes required to resolve the dispute. Had Jayna's therapist more carefully considered the impact of Jayna's 8 years of mood symptoms and recognized how these symptoms had delayed her social and emotional development, she might have selected interpersonal deficits as the problem area and focused more on helping Jayna to move gradually toward a more adult self-concept. Undoubtedly, this approach would have required a great deal more subtlety than the behavioral approach taken to the role dispute with her mother, but in the end it might have led to less frustration for both Jayna and her therapist.

Positive feelings about a patient or too close an identification with the patient's circumstances can also inhibit treatment progress. The following case example illustrates this potential pitfall.

CASE EXAMPLE

Eleni, a doctoral candidate in psychology at a local university, was diagnosed with bipolar disorder following a trip to visit her extended family in Greece over the Christmas holiday. Eleni returned to the United States in a manic state, believing she was the goddess Aphrodite incarnate and planning to spread "love and peace" throughout the world. She was hospitalized briefly and discharged to the care of a psychiatrist and an IPSRT therapist. The therapist immediately liked Eleni. She was a bright, engaging individual with a good sense of humor and an appreciation for the ironies of being diagnosed with bipolar disorder while working on a PhD in psychology. Eleni was able to quickly return to her studies and seemed to be doing very well on lithium alone. Sessions with Eleni focused on helping her rearrange her work habits to promote regular sleep and identifying priorities so that she could eliminate unnecessary activities, thereby reducing stimulation. Eleni often regaled her therapist with stories of departmental politics and scandals, information that her therapist secretly enjoyed because she had graduated from the same doctoral program several years before. As Eleni's comprehensive exams approached, she began to study more and sleep less. Although the therapist cautioned her against disrupting her social rhythms, she was highly sympathetic to Eleni's need to prepare for her exams.

The night before she was to take her exams, Eleni was brought to the emergency room by her roommate, who had found her disorganized and agitated in the dormitory study room at 3 o'clock in the morning. In retrospect, the therapist felt that she had underestimated the potential seriousness of Eleni's behaviors because of an overidentification with the patient and her circumstances.

Had Eleni's therapist not overidentified with this appealing patient, she would have been able to be more cautionary with her. She also would have tried to engage the treating psychiatrist in warning Eleni about the dangers of her current lifestyle. In Eleni's case, she neglected to do so because of her ability to understand—from her own experience as a graduate student—the contingencies to which Eleni was responding. What she neglected to think about was the extent to which her patient's bipolar disorder necessitated finding an entirely different way to respond to those contingencies than that she had used herself as a grad student. Indeed, she might even have talked with Eleni about the possibility of discussing some special considerations relative to her comps, given her disability. For example, Eleni might have requested that her comps be divided into two or three testing sessions, separated by several weeks, in order to give her time to study for each one while still maintaining regular social rhythms and getting adequate sleep each night. Under the Americans with Disabilities Act she would have been entitled to such an accommodation. Unfortunately, though, this never occurred to Eleni's overidentified clinician.

Another crucial aspect of working with patients with bipolar disorder is flexibility. Psychotherapists trained in IPSRT have an overall focus for the treatment at any point in time and often a specific plan for upcoming sessions. Patients who have been depressed during most of the treatment may experience a mood change to a manic state during the week prior to a session, or vice versa. In this case, the therapist will be forced to think on his or her feet, quickly switching foci and strategies. It is important for therapists to assess subtle changes, as well, and make the necessary interventions and take the necessary precautions as a result of any changes they observe. It is very important that IPSRT therapists be skilled in identifying major and minor shifts in moods that a particular patient brings to treatment. Often patients are not aware of their subtle hypomanic symptoms. The therapist cannot be intimidated by patients (who can be irritable and intimidating when their moods are elevated) or frightened to point out these changes.

IS THIS A CASE OF POOR OUTCOME
OR INAPPROPRIATE EXPECTATIONS?

When evaluating sources of treatment difficulty or "poor" outcome, it is also important to be clear in your own mind about what kinds of outcomes can and should be targeted. In some cases, what appears to be a poor outcome can, in fact, reflect unrealistic expectations for the pace of change. As noted in earlier chapters, particularly among patients with interpersonal deficits, the time course for change may be much longer than might be predicted on this basis of the patient's superficial social skills, intelligence, and energy level. This can be an especially vexing problem for therapists when family members are unable to accept the pace of change in their loved one or when their expectations for change exceed those of the therapist. The solution in these cases may be to adjust one's expectations (and/or the patient's expectations) and help the patient manage the frustrations of an illness that is, at times, quite limiting.

CASE EXAMPLE

Tom was a 25-year-old graduate student in visual arts who had developed his first manic episode after hanging his first solo show in graduate school. The mania led to hospitalization and was followed by a severe and protracted depression that led him to drop out of graduate school. When he entered psychotherapy, he was living at home and was completely isolated. He had no social contacts other than his parents and two younger siblings. Tom was very traumatized by the experience of a psychotic mania and his unremitting depression. His goal was to achieve mood stability, with a plan to reassess his career goals once his mood was back to "normal." His parents, however, were narcissistically invested in their son's artistic career and were unable to understand why he was unable to resume his painting. They repeatedly mentioned to the patient and the therapist that they had cleared space in the basement for Tom to use as a studio and had been in touch with the graduate program which, they assured both patient and therapist, was eager to take him back. Tom seemed to make little progress in the first months of treatment. It eventually became apparent that the pressure put on him by his parents was contributing to Tom's failure to improve. The therapist spent several sessions with Tom's parents, educating them about the expectable course of bipolar disorder and the importance of allowing Tom to determine the conditions under which he returned to his artwork. Receptive to the therapist's suggestions, the parents reduced their expectations and joined a support group as a means of expressing (and containing) their frustration with their son. Without the constant pressure from his parents, Tom felt better able to explore honestly his own needs and goals. Over time, he achieved a remarkably stable mood and very slowly began to reengage in his artwork. Two and a half years after the initial mania, Tom took a job teaching art in an elementary school. He hoped to return to his own artwork some day, but felt that, for now, a "regular" job was more in keeping with his goal of mood stability than the exciting but potentially destabilizing path of pursuing his own career in the art world. Tom's parents were surprisingly supportive of his decision.

Sometimes inappropriate expectations come not from the patient, his family, or his friends, but from the therapist. Poor treatment attendance is often a sign that this is the case, a sign to which therapists should pay close attention.

CASE EXAMPLE

Jeff was a 33-year-old male with a long history of untreated bipolar disorder when he entered IPRST. As he began psychotherapy, he was experiencing his first period of sustained euthymic mood since early adolescence. Despite his obviously high intelligence, he had little to show in the way of educational or occupational attainment. Raised in a severely abusive family characterized by psychopathology and drug addiction in many family members, Jeff had no close family relationships and few friends. He had dropped out of high school at 17 and left home, drifting from job to job and town to town, often forming relationships in which he ended up feeling used, just the way he had felt used by his even more dysfunctional family members. He had subsequently obtained a general equivalency diploma, but had never received any formal post-high school education. Once he realized that many of his difficulties after leaving home could be explained by his untreated bipolar disorder, Jeff's goal for himself became to obtain a college degree. His dream was to get a steady full-time job as a computer graphic artist, something for which he had already evidenced a fair degree of talent. Jeff's only interpersonal goal was to stay out of destructive relationships. He was completely focused on getting an education and had convinced himself that friends would be, at best, a distraction and a romance would be a disaster. His therapist, however, felt that it would be important to his quality of life to bring some social relationships into his life. At that time, Jeff had no real relationships with others beyond superficial relationships with coworkers at the Kinko's where he was employed. The therapist noted, however, that any time she broached the subject of reuniting with family members or expanding Jeff's social circle, he would cancel the next appointment and be difficult to track down for several weeks. The third time this happened, the therapist confronted Jeff directly on this issue. He acknowledged that he had been very upset by the discussion of his need for interpersonal relationships. Indeed, he had cried the whole way home from their previous session and his mood was down for several days thereafter. He admitted that he was just too frightened of being involved with people to address this issue. He made it clear that as far as he was concerned, his focus needed to be on doing well in his college studies, obtaining his degree, and securing the kind of steady employment he had sought for so long. Once Jeff's therapist was able to acknowledge that her goals for him were technically appropriate but premature, and once she was able to keep the therapy focused on Jeff's transition to full-time school and academic success, his therapy attendance became regular and his mood continued to stabilize further.

COMPLICATIONS AND COMORBIDITIES: WHEN YOUR SKILL SET MAY NOT BE ENOUGH

There are some patients who will fail to improve despite optimal treatment. This experience can be very demoralizing for a therapist. It is important to remember, however, that this is even more demoralizing for the patient. As the therapist you can play an important role in offering your patient support through the course of illness, while continuing to offer hope about the possibility of a new treatment becoming available to treat this illness. There are also times when you will have to acknowledge that additional therapy skills are needed that you do not possess.

CASE EXAMPLE

Mannie was a 41-year-old male with a 21-year history of bipolar disorder. Although he was a very bright man and had matriculated at a prestigious college, he had dropped out in the middle of his sophomore year following an amphetamine-induced mania. Mannie continued to struggle with his illness over the next 20 years. At times, he would seem to improve enough to think about looking for a job, but then he would quickly slide back into a depression. He continued to struggle with substance abuse, intermittently using cocaine and methamphetamine to counteract his grinding depression. Bouts of heavy substance abuse often led to decreased sleep, medication noncompliance, and hospitalization. Very little seemed to change for Mannie over time. He often felt like giving up and, since turning 40, had frequent suicidal thoughts: "My life is a waste," he would say at each session. His therapist provided a supportive environment for Mannie to express his feelings. He encouraged Mannie to mourn the lost healthy self while helping him to set modest goals for himself in the short term. He supported Mannie's efforts to seek consultation from a renowned pharmacologist and reminded him that his dual problems—bipolar disorder and substance abuse—might be especially difficult, but not impossible, to treat. Perhaps most important, he acknowledged that although he could help Mannie with his bipolar symptoms, his expertise did not extend to substance abuse treatment. Although Mannie initially felt even more demoralized at the thought that he needed three clinicians to treat his illness, his IPSRT therapist was finally able to convince him that this three-pronged approach might finally give him the stability he had sought for so long.

At times, modifications in the pharmacotherapy, the psychotherapy, or other aspects of the treatment intervention can make a substantial difference in outcome. Sometimes these will be minor adjustments in the focus of your psychosocial intervention, or even a complete shift in the interpersonal problem area being focused upon. At other times, there will be minor or complete changes in the patient's pharmacotherapy. At still other times, there will be changes in the therapeutic relationship itself or in your attitude toward your patient. If all possible sources of difficulty in the treatment have been explored and the outcome remains below your expectations, it may be necessary to acknowledge that in some cases of bipolar disorder even maintaining the status quo and preventing further deterioration is a small victory.

FOURTEEN

Tapering or Concluding Treatment

As stated explicitly in earlier chapters, we are ambivalent about the question of concluding treatment in patients who suffer from what is almost always a lifelong condition. On one hand, having been thoroughly schooled in the tradition of the short-term psychotherapies, we understand the value of focused, goal-oriented treatment that remains directed to the patient's present problems and does not foster dependency. On the other hand, taking as we do a chronic disease management perspective in our treatment of bipolar disorder, we argue that there may well be cases in which true termination should never take place.

Indeed, my initial prototype for IPSRT grew out of my work with a woman by the name of Lois who was referred to me more than two decades ago. She suffers from a severe form of bipolar I disorder, complicated by co-occurring panic disorder, not an unusual combination. When Lois first came to see me, she had a history of multiple severe suicide attempts, had been hospitalized many times, at one point for more than a year. That episode was brought to an end only when her father had her removed from the hospital, where she was being allowed to linger in an essentially catatonic state as the unit's 65-pound "hopeless case," a term she often heard the hospital staff use to describe her. Her father put her in the hands of a courageous psychiatrist who, despite his psychoanalytic training, was willing to give her electroconvulsive therapy (ECT). She improved rapidly and dramatically as a result of the ECT treatments and was able to return home within a matter of weeks. Still, she remained chronically anxious, moderately depressed, and severely impaired in her functioning. When her new psychiatrist despaired of ever bringing her into full remission, he suggested that she seek more state-of-the-art treatment. At his recommendation, she subsequently spent more than 7 months in the inpatient unit of the National Institute of Mental Health Clinical Center in the hope that it would find some treatment that would give her the mood stability she so desperately wanted. She returned home marginally better, largely thanks to massive doses of neuroleptic that relieved her terrible panic and anxiety. But she was still determined that she could improve further and return to something like normal functioning. She had read about cognitive therapy in *Reader's Digest* and thought that maybe a more behavioral approach to her treatment would help. Her psychiatrist agreed that it was worth a try.

When she first appeared in my office, her attire was clean but otherwise her appearance was that of someone who simply did not care about herself. She reported rarely leaving her apartment except to visit her one close friend. She was still unemployed, despite very high intelligence and a history of successful functioning as a technical writer. Her economic circumstances were quite precarious.

She quickly caught on to the social rhythm and behavioral activation aspects of the treatment. With encouragement and validation that she deserved to do so, she began paying more attention to her appearance, taking some of her beautiful old work attire out from the depths of her closet and having her hair cut professionally for the first time in many years. She began to reconnect with her formerly large circle of friends.

After approximately 4 months of treatment with what was embryonic social rhythm therapy, she had made modest, but clear gains in her depressive symptoms and functioning. She was beginning to enjoy her life a tiny bit.

At that point, going by the short-term therapy "book," I began to discuss termination and attempted to reduce the frequency of therapy sessions with an eye toward ending her treatment after a total of 20 or so sessions. Somehow, each time I would schedule a session 2 weeks hence, a crisis intervened: Her precious dog would become ill, her father's nursing home would threaten to discharge him, and so forth. The net result was that we continued to see one another on a more or less weekly basis for the next 3 or 4 months. At the end of that time, with her functioning continuing to improve, her mood remaining stable for one of the longest periods since the onset of her illness, I began to question the value of terminating treatment with Lois. The goal was to keep her well, and this treatment seemed to be doing that. Did she know more than I did about what it would take to sustain her first long remission in more than a decade?

ONGOING MAINTENANCE TREATMENT WITH IPSRT

I have continued to see Lois on a two- to three-session-per-month basis since that time. It has now been more than 22 years. During that time, she has evidenced steady improvement in her functioning. She now boasts a wide circle of highly supportive friends whom she, in turn, has supported in a number of important ways over this period of time. For several years, she ran her own private baking business, which she called "Manna," because she believed her ability to manage such a venture was a gift from heaven. She volunteered at the art museum and at a huge soup kitchen in her neighborhood, cooking meals for homeless people, who reminded her each week of what her own fate might have been.

More recently, using the strategies and tactics of *grief for the lost healthy self*, she has been able to cope well with very significant changes in her health, including the loss of most of her vision. Perhaps most important, she has been hospitalized only three times in the course of these 22 years and has never made another suicide attempt.

There are some patients whose bipolar illness is so severe that as long as they (or the government) are able to pay for ongoing treatment, termination simply makes no sense. Had Lois's course of illness continued as it was when I first saw her, at a minimum she would have cost the government hundreds of thousands of dollars in hospital charges, to say nothing of her personal suffering if she had survived these 22 years without a successful suicide attempt.

We do not think to question the ongoing involvement in treatment of a patient with severe life-threatening asthma, heart disease, or diabetes. Indeed, we encourage such patients to remain in constant contact with their clinicians and to be monitored on a very regular basis for progression of their disease. Bipolar illness is also a life-threatening disease, one for which lifelong psychotherapy, as well as pharmacotherapy may be indicated.

TERMINATING IPSRT

There are, however, patients whose bipolar illness is not so severe and who, for personal or practical reasons, are candidates for a shorter-term therapy approach. Probably the minimum amount of time for an adequate IPSRT intervention is 20–24 sessions, spaced over something like 5–8 months. In the case of a patient who is functioning well, who does not have a past history of severe, damaging psychotic episodes or suicide attempts, and who has a relatively supportive social network, it is reasonable to terminate IPSRT, with the proviso that the patient can return to treatment should he or she become symptomatic again or feel the need for some additional coaching with respect to either rhythm stability or interpersonal problems. Other patients may *need* to terminate treatment because of relocation or an inability to pay for further therapy. In all such cases, termination is ideally planned well in advance. The last several sessions are then spent reviewing the progress that patient has made and discussing strategies for relapse prevention.

In the process of termination, you will probably find it useful to return to the illness history timeline developed at the beginning of treatment. It is often helpful to patients to extend that timeline through to the present day as you are terminating treatment, asking the patient to focus on the improvements that he or she feels have occurred and on any goals the patient may have for further improvement in either the rhythm stability or the interpersonal arena. The same kind of review of the illness history timeline can be helpful at key points earlier in therapy, such as at the transition from acute to maintenance treatment or at the end of the first 6 months or first year of maintenance therapy. It can also be helpful at the time of a relapse or recurrence to help both you and your patient understand what might have gone wrong and to see it in this graphical way.

Because, in the ideal case, IPSRT treatment will have lasted many months, this review of illness history before and since engagement in IPSRT should yield a picture of numerous gains in patients who have worked hard in the therapy. Keep in mind, however, that what we once thought of as a "good prognosis" condition often proves to be a deteriorative one, especially for those patients who experience the cognitive impairment that we now understand is associated with bipolar I disorder. For older patients with histories of severe illness, just maintaining themselves at the level at which they entered treatment can sometimes be considered a real victory. Particularly when such patients have seen family members or fellow patients deteriorate substantially as a result of bipolar illness, your pointing out that maintaining status quo can be considered a major accomplishment can be a very therapeutic intervention.

CASE EXAMPLE

For Steve, whose case is described earlier in Chapters 6 and 9, it took a little more than 2 years to recover functionally, despite the absence of overt depressive or hypomanic symptoms. After about a year of treatment, he was ready to begin looking for employment again, but found that his age was working against him. He realized, however, that the only reason he had been terminated from his former government job was his outrageous behavior while manic. Finally, with 18 months of stability under his belt and a good understanding of his rights, he decided to sue the government for reinstatement. With the support of his therapist and his pharmacotherapist, who were both convinced that he was more than ready and capable to return to his former position, he succeeded in getting his job back. This would mean, however, leaving the city and returning to his former home in a little over 3 months' time. Steve's therapist used their last four sessions to review his illness history timeline. She reviewed the slow, but steady progress he had made during treatment and reassured him of his readiness to return to the very stimulating environment in which he had worked. She reviewed again, in minute detail, the circumstances surrounding and the early warning signs (which he had missed) of his last two manic episodes. She and Steve discussed what he would need to do to avoid such circumstances: He could probably manage his job quite well, but was likely better off staying away from the political organizing and campaigning he had done in the past. He would need to lead a somewhat quieter life. They discussed what challenges there might be to maintaining stable social rhythms and whether and how he should reconnect with his old friends.

A key part of the process of termination is ensuring the ongoing management of your patient's pharmacological treatment. If you have been working as part of a treatment team, terminating with you may mean that your patient must also leave his or her pharmacotherapist. In this case, you will want to be certain that the pharmacological treatment the patient is entering is of good quality. Under the best circumstances, a change in the patient's pharmacotherapist and your termination of treatment would not occur simultaneously. Rather, it would be good to be able to follow your patient for a couple of months after making the transition to the new pharmacotherapist. When such a shift is necessitated by relocation, this may not be possible, but phone contact can be maintained, with complete termination occurring only after you are satisfied that the patient has made a good connection to the new pharmacotherapist.

Because IPSRT is not yet a widely diffused treatment, a patient's relocation to another city before treatment is complete can represent a particular termination challenge. Here, again, you want first to try to ensure the best possible pharmacotherapy for your patient and, if possible, transfer to a qualified psychotherapist. The second objective may prove to be the much greater challenge. In all probability, the best you can hope for is to find someone with a present-oriented, problem-focused approach to treatment who has had experience in working with patients who suffer from bipolar disorder. You will want to discuss with your patient how he or she plans to describe IPSRT to the new therapist, with particular emphasis on helping him or her to think about and communicate what has been most helpful about IPSRT. It undoubtedly will also be helpful if you can share directly with your patient's future therapist something about the kind of treatment the patient has been receiving. The availability of this book should aid in that process.

MAINTAINING CONTACT AFTER TERMINATION

At the outset of our work in IPSRT, maintaining contact after termination was not a topic we would have thought to address in this book; however, again, we have learned much from our patients. What we have observed is that patients who are able to remain stable and do not need our clinical attention, nonetheless want us to be aware of how they are doing. Indeed, that stability represents not just their triumph, but the triumph of the treatment approach, and they seem to want to let us know that it continues to work for them. We typically hear from these patients on something like an annual basis, and we always respond, saying how pleased we are that things continue to go well.

Tad (discussed in Chapter 1) writes at the close of each school year, telling us with his wry Southern wit about the many funny things his students did that year, the competitions they have won, and why next year's classes can't possibly compete with this year's crop. He tells us how tolerant his principal is of his "creative" curriculum and how supportive his mom continues to be. He tells us what his plans are for the summer, always reassuring us that he will stay in his routine and thanking us, yet again, for teaching him how he needed to live his life if he wanted to stay well.

Jill (also discussed in Chapter 1) doesn't write, but stops by the clinic, sometimes with her boys, whenever she is in town. She has moved to Seattle and, although it means that the boys don't get to see their father as much as she would like, it has meant that she has the support of her brother and sister-in-law and the boys have their cousins to run with. All you have to do is spend a few minutes with her sons to know how well Jill is doing: They are full of spirit and enthusiasm, but calm, well mannered, and articulate. It is a delight to spend time with them. It is also a delight to see how well all three of them have done. With more than a decade of stability under her belt and her younger son entering high school, Jill is thinking about looking for a teaching job, maybe at a junior college in her area. Although it's been years since they've seen one another regularly, she still would like to know what her IPSRT therapist thinks of the idea.

Appendices

APPENDIX 1. Social Rhythm Metric–II—Five-Item Version (SRM-II-5)

Directions:

Date (week of): _____

- Write the **ideal target time** you would **like** to do these daily activities.
- Record the **time** you **actually** did the activity each day.
- Record the **people** involved in the activity: 0 = Alone; 1 = Others present; 2 = Others actively involved; 3 = Others very stimulating

Activity	Target time	Sunday		Monday		Tuesday		Wednesday		Thursday		Friday		Saturday	
		Time	People	Time	People	Time	People	Time	People	Time	People	Time	People	Time	People
Out of bed															
First contact with other person															
Start work/school/ volunteer/family care															
Dinner															
To bed															
Rate MOOD each day from –5 to +5: –5 = very depressed +5 = very elated															

From *Treating Bipolar Disorder: A Clinician's Guide to Interpersonal Social Rhythm Therapy* by Ellen Frank. Copyright 2005 by The Guilford Press. Permission to photocopy this appendix is granted to purchasers of this book for personal use only (see copyright page for details).

APPENDIX 2. Score Calculation Instructions for the SRM-II-5

Basically, the scoring algorithm for the SRM-II-5 is the same as for the SRM-II-17 (see Appendix 4). Let us take a simple example to explain the process for the SRM-II-5:

Suppose this is what we see when we look at a person's diary for the 7 days of the week. For 5 days the person got up, usually at or near 6:00 A.M., but on 2 days it was 8:00 A.M, which is more than 45 minutes from 6:00 A.M., so the hits for "out of bed" were 5. For first contact with another person, he phoned his mother every morning at 7:00 A.M., except on 2 days when he got up late and phoned her after 9:00 A.M., and on 1 day when his mother was out of town visiting a friend when he did not call her at all and spent the day alone at home. Then first contact has a hit score of 4. For 5 days he went to the office and was there within 45 minutes of 7:30 A.M., so the hit score for "start work" is 5. Dinner is very variable for our person: the usual time is 8:15 P.M., but only twice this particular week was his dinner time within 45 minutes of 8:15. Dinner has a hit score of 2. At the end of each day, he went to bed at 10:30 usually, but on 1 night it was after midnight. "To bed" then has a hit score of 6. So for the five events, our person's SRM score is (5 + 4 + 6 + 2 + 6)/5, which is 4.6.

For full score calculation instructions for the Social Rhythm Metric—17-item version, see Appendix 4.

From *Treating Bipolar Disorder: A Clinician's Guide to Interpersonal Social Rhythm Therapy* by Ellen Frank. Copyright 2005 by The Guilford Press. Permission to photocopy this appendix is granted to purchasers of this book for personal use only (see copyright page for details).

APPENDIX 3. Social Rhythm Metric–II—17-Item Version (SRM-II-17)

Name: _____   Date: __ __/__ __/__ __
                                                             m m d d y y

Please Fill This Out at the End of the Day

Day of Week: _____

ACTIVITY	TIME	A.M. or P.M.	M	T	W	Th	F	Sa	Su
PEOPLE 0 = Alone, 1 = Others just present, 2 = Others actively involved, 3 = Others very stimulating									
OUT OF BED	Earlier								
	Exact earlier time								
midpoint of your normal range									
	Later								
	Exact later time								
	Check if did not do								

(cont.)

From *Treating Bipolar Disorder: A Clinician's Guide to Interpersonal Social Rhythm Therapy* by Ellen Frank. Copyright 2005 by The Guilford Press. Permission to photocopy this appendix is granted to purchasers of this book for personal use only (see copyright page for details).

		A.M.	**DAY OF WEEK**						
PEOPLE 0 = Alone	1 = Others just present	2 = Others actively involved	3 = Others very stimulating						

ACTIVITY	TIME	A.M. or P.M.	M	T	W	Th	F	Sa	Su
FIRST CONTACT (IN PERSON OR BY PHONE) WITH ANOTHER PERSON	Earlier								
	Exact earlier time								
midpoint of your normal range →									
	Later								
	Exact later time								
	Check if did not do								
HAVE MORNING BEVERAGE	Earlier								
	Exact earlier time								
midpoint of your normal range →									
	Later								
	Exact later time								
	Check if did not do								

(cont.)

		A.M. or P.M.	DAY OF WEEK						
PEOPLE 0 = Alone 1 = Others just present 2 = Others actively involved 3 = Others very stimulating									
ACTIVITY	**TIME**		**M**	**T**	**W**	**Th**	**F**	**Sa**	**Su**
HAVE BREAKFAST	Earlier								
	Exact earlier time								
midpoint of your normal range →									
	Later								
	Exact later time								
	Check if did not do								

(cont.)

		A.M. or P.M.	DAY OF WEEK						
PEOPLE 0 = Alone 1 = Others just present 2 = Others actively involved 3 = Others very stimulating									
ACTIVITY	**TIME**		**M**	**T**	**W**	**Th**	**F**	**Sa**	**Su**
GO OUTSIDE FOR THE FIRST TIME	Earlier								
	Exact earlier time								
midpoint of your normal range →									
	Later								
	Exact later time								
	Check if did not do								

(cont.)

		A.M. or P.M.	DAY OF WEEK						
PEOPLE 0 = Alone 1 = Others just present 2 = Others actively involved 3 = Others very stimulating									
ACTIVITY	**TIME**		**M**	**T**	**W**	**Th**	**F**	**Sa**	**Su**
START WORK, SCHOOL, HOUSEWORK, VOLUNTEER ACTIVITIES, CHILD OR FAMILY CARE	Earlier								
	Exact earlier time								
midpoint of your normal range →									
	Later								
	Exact later time								
	Check if did not do								
HAVE LUNCH	Earlier								
	Exact earlier time								
midpoint of your normal range →									
	Later								
	Exact later time								
	Check if did not do								

(cont.)

		A.M. or P.M.	DAY OF WEEK						
			PEOPLE 0 = Alone 1 = Others just present 2 = Others actively involved 3 = Others very stimulating						
ACTIVITY	TIME		M	T	W	Th	F	Sa	Su
TAKE AN AFTERNOON NAP	Earlier								
	Exact earlier time								
midpoint of your normal range									
	Later								
	Exact later time								
	Check if did not do								
HAVE DINNER	Earlier								
	Exact earlier time								
midpoint of your normal range									
	Later								
	Exact later time								
	Check if did not do								

(cont.)

171

		A.M. or P.M.	DAY OF WEEK						
PEOPLE 0 = Alone 1 = Others just present 2 = Others actively involved 3 = Others very stimulating									
ACTIVITY	**TIME**		**M**	**T**	**W**	**Th**	**F**	**Sa**	**Su**
PHYSICAL EXERCISE	Earlier								
	Exact earlier time								
midpoint of your normal → range									
	Later								
	Exact later time								
	Check if did not do								

(cont.)

		A.M. or P.M.	DAY OF WEEK						
PEOPLE 0 = Alone 1 = Others just present 2 = Others actively involved 3 = Others very stimulating									
ACTIVITY	**TIME**		**M**	**T**	**W**	**Th**	**F**	**Sa**	**Su**
HAVE AN EVENING SNACK/DRINK	Earlier								
	Exact earlier time								
midpoint of your normal → range									
	Later								
	Exact later time								
	Check if did not do								
WATCH EVENING TV NEWS PROGRAM	Earlier								
	Exact earlier time								
midpoint of your normal → range									
	Later								
	Exact later time								
	Check if did not do								

(cont.)

			PEOPLE 0 = Alone 1 = Others just present 2 = Others actively involved 3 = Others very stimulating						
ACTIVITY	**TIME**	**A.M. or P.M.**	**DAY OF WEEK**						
			M	**T**	**W**	**Th**	**F**	**Sa**	**Su**
WATCH ANOTHER TV PROGRAM	Earlier								
	Exact earlier time								
midpoint of your normal → range									
	Later								
	Exact later time								
	Check if did not do								

(cont.)

ACTIVITY	TIME	A.M. or P.M.	PEOPLE 0 = Alone 1 = Others just present 2 = Others actively involved 3 = Others very stimulating						
			DAY OF WEEK						
			M	T	W	Th	F	Sa	Su
ACTIVITY A	Earlier								
	Exact earlier time								
midpoint of your normal range →									
	Later								
	Exact later time								
	Check if did not do								

(cont.)

		A.M. or P.M.	DAY OF WEEK						
			PEOPLE 0 = Alone 1 = Others just present 2 = Others actively involved 3 = Others very stimulating						
ACTIVITY	**TIME**		**M**	**T**	**W**	**Th**	**F**	**Sa**	**Su**
ACTIVITY B	Earlier								
	Exact earlier time								
midpoint of your normal → range									
	Later								
	Exact later time								
	Check if did not do								

(cont.)

		A.M. or P.M.	DAY OF WEEK						
			PEOPLE 0 = Alone 1 = Others just present 2 = Others actively involved 3 = Others very stimulating						
ACTIVITY	**TIME**	**A.M. or P.M.**	**M**	**T**	**W**	**Th**	**F**	**Sa**	**Su**
RETURN HOME (LAST TIME)	Earlier								
	Exact earlier time								
midpoint of your normal range →									
	Later								
	Exact later time								
	Check if did not do								

(cont.)

		A.M. or P.M.	DAY OF WEEK						
PEOPLE 0 = Alone 1 = Others just present 2 = Others actively involved 3 = Others very stimulating									
ACTIVITY	**TIME**		**M**	**T**	**W**	**Th**	**F**	**Sa**	**Su**
GO TO BED	Earlier								
	Exact earlier time								
midpoint of your normal range →									
	Later								
	Exact later time								
	Check if did not do								

MOOD RATING											**DAY OF WEEK**
				Scale							
−5	−4	−3	−2	−1	0	+1	+2	+3	+4	+5	
very depressed					normal					very elated	

APPENDIX 4. Score Calculation Instructions for the SRM-II-17

Note: When used for research purposes, the SRM-II-17 is scored according to the following instructions; however, it is not necessary to score the SRM-II-17 to use it as a clinical monitoring device.

ALGORITHM (NARRATIVE) FOR CALCULATING SCORES ON THE SRM-II-17

1. Compute the average time each activity was performed. For example, let us imagine that a patient performed Activity A (which, for her, was walking her dog) at the following times:

   6:00 A.M.   On day #1
   5:50 A.M.   On day #2
   8:01 A.M.   On day #3
   7:55 A.M.   On day #4
   5:45 A.M.   On day #5
   5:50 A.M.   On day #6
   5:50 A.M.   On day #7

   The average time for Activity A is 6:27 A.M.; the standard deviation (*SD*) is 62 minutes.

2. Compute the minimum and maximum time range to determine outliers. (Outliers are activity times that fall outside 1.5 *SD* from the mean.)

   Formulas are:
   MINTIME = AVERAGE TIME − (1.5* *SD*)
   MAXTIME = AVERAGE TIME + (1.5* *SD*)

   Substituting values yields:
   MINTIME = 6:27 − (93 minutes) = 4:54
   MAXTIME = 6:27 + (93 minutes) = 8:00

   Therefore, nonoutlier data fall within this range:
   MINTIME < TIME < MAXTIME

   Or, in this example:
   4:54 < TIME < 8:00

3. Using the raw data from step 1, we can see that all the times fall within this range except for 8:01 (occurring on day #3). This time, 8:01 A.M., is considered an outlier.

4. Now, we have only nonoutlier data for 6 days.

   6:00 A.M.   On day #1
   5:50 A.M.   On day #2
   7:55 A.M.   On day #4
   5:45 A.M.   On day #5
   5:50 A.M.   On day #7

5. Recompute the mean using only nonoutlier data; this is the habitual time. For this example, the habitual time is 6:12 A.M..

(cont.)

From *Treating Bipolar Disorder: A Clinician's Guide to Interpersonal Social Rhythm Therapy* by Ellen Frank. Copyright 2005 by The Guilford Press. Permission to photocopy this appendix is granted to purchasers of this book for personal use only (see copyright page for details).

6. Recombine the nonoutlier data and the outlier data to determine hits. A "hit" is an activity time that occurs within 45 minutes of the habitual time.

   Formulas are:

   > MINIMUM TIME FOR HIT = NEW MEAN = 45 minutes
   > MAXIMUM TIME FOR HIT = NEW MEAN = 45 minutes

   Substituting our values, we get:

   > MINHIT = 6:12 − 45 minutes = 5:27 A.M.
   > MAXHIT = 6:12 + 45 minutes = 6:57 A.M.

   Therefore, a time is considered a "hit" if it falls between 5:27 A.M. and 6:57 A.M. (MINHIT < TIME < MAXHIT).

   Using all of the data:

6:00 A.M.	On day #1
5:50 A.M.	On day #2
8:01 A.M.	On day #3
7:55 A.M.	On day #4
5:45 A.M.	On day #5
5:50 A.M.	On day #6
5:50 A.M.	On day #7

   We see that all of the activity times fell within this range except 8:01 A.M. and 7:55 A.M. (occurring on day #3 and day #4, respectively). Therefore, we can say that for Activity A, the person had:

   a. 7 days with a possible hit
   b. 5 hits across those 7 days

7. Using all 17 activities, select activities that occurred at least 3 times per week (Activity A would be included because the person had 7 days of data).

8. Calculate the number of activities occurring at least 3 times/week and the total number of hits for those activities.

   For example: Out of 17 activities, 5 of them occurred at least 3 times/week ($n = 5$):

Activity	Days with a possible hit	Hits across those days
1	5	4
2	7	5
4	3	1
11	4	2
17	7	7
	$n = 5$	Total 19

9. The Social Rhythm Metric II (SRM-II) score is defined as:

   $$\text{SRM-II-17 score} = \frac{\text{Total number of hits for activities that occurred GE 3 times/week}}{\text{Number of activities occurring at least 3 times/week } (n)}$$

   (cont.)

Score Calculation Instructions for the SRM-II-17 (page 3 of 3)

Using the data values in step 8,

SRM-II score = 19/5 = 3.8

SCORING: FLOW DIAGRAM FOR SRM-II-17 ALGORITHM*

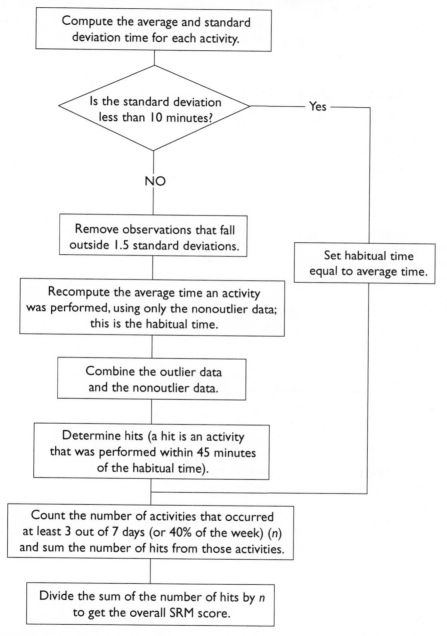

From Monk, Kupfer, Frank, and Ritenour (1991). (See Section III.) Copyright 1991 by Elsevier Inc. Adapted by permission.

An Interview Guide for the Interpersonal Inventory

Name: _____

Date: _____

NOTE: Much of the information needed to complete the interpersonal inventory is likely to emerge as you take the history of the patient's illness. The various sections of this interview guide are intended to be used to fill in gaps in your knowledge following completion of the illness history timeline.

SECTION A—CLOSE RELATIONSHIPS

Notes

A1	***Who would you say are the important people in your life right now? Do you have close relationships?***	
	If yes, investigate the quality of these relationships.	
	Who are the people closest to you? Family members? Friends? Lover? Coworkers? Others?	
	Do you talk openly about personal problems with any of these people? Which ones?	
	If the patient denies having anyone to whom he or she is close right now, go to Sections A3 and A4.	

(cont.)

From *Treating Bipolar Disorder: A Clinician's Guide to Interpersonal Social Rhythm Therapy* by Ellen Frank. Copyright 2005 by The Guilford Press. Permission to photocopy this appendix is granted to purchasers of this book for personal use only (see copyright page for details).

Notes

A2	Ask the following about each important person in the patient's current life:	
I.	Can you ask for his/her help when you have problems?	
2.	Do you trust him/her and feel understood?	
3.	Do you feel he/she trusts you and confides in you as well?	
4.	How does your relationship with him/her make you feel?	
5.	What are the positive and negative aspects of this relationship?	
6.	Do you think that your illness has had an impact on your relationship? In what way?	
7.	Is there anything you'd like to be different in this relationship, anything you'd like to change in yourself and/or in the other person in order to make the relationship better?	
8.	How often do you see or talk to him/her?	
9.	What sorts of things do you do together?	
A3	*Have you had close relationships in the past? When was that?*	

(cont.)

Notes

A4	***Ask the following about each important person in the patient's earlier life:***	
1.	How did you get along with him/her?	
2.	Why did this relationship end?	
3.	Do you feel that you have problems getting close to people?	
4.	Do you find it difficult to keep close relationships once you make them?	
5.	Do you have problems knowing what to do in a relationship once you go beyond first meeting the person?	
6.	Did you make any new friends in this past year?	
7.	Do you enjoy close relationships when you have them?	
8.	Do you miss having or would you like to have close relationships?	
9.	Do you feel lonely?	
10.	Do you feel bored?	
11.	How often do you go out?	
	What sorts of things do you enjoy doing?	
	Do you do them alone or with someone else (who)?	

(cont.)

		Notes
12.	Has your social life been more active in the past?	
13.	Would you like your social life to be more active?	

SECTION B—IDENTIFICATION OF OTHER PROBLEM AREAS

		Notes
B1	***Now, I'd like you to think back to the time when this depression (or mania) began . . .***	
1.	Did someone you care about die?	
2.	Was it the anniversary of someone's death around the time your depression began?	
3.	Were you thinking a lot about someone who died around the time your depression began?	
4.	Were you having problems at home with your spouse or partner?	
5.	Were you having problems with your children?	
6.	Were you having problems with your parents?	
7.	Were you having problems with your brothers or sisters?	
8.	Were you having problems with your in-laws?	
9.	Were you having problems at work?	
10.	Were you having problems with your friends?	

(cont.)

Notes

11.	Were you having problems with others?	
12.	Were there more arguments with family or friends?	
13.	Were you disappointed in a love relationship?	
14.	Did you begin to have problems in your marriage?	
15.	Were you going through a divorce or separation?	
16.	Did your children leave home?	
17.	Did you take a new job?	
18.	Did you lose a job?	
19.	Did you get promoted?	
20.	Did you retire?	
21.	Did you start school?	
22.	Did you graduate?	
23.	Did you move?	
24.	Did someone move in with you?	
25.	Did you start living alone?	
26.	Did you have financial problems?	

(cont.)

Notes

27.	Did you become ill?	
28.	Was there a serious illness in your family?	
29.	Were you worried about any relatives or friends for another reason?	
30.	Did you lose contact with someone important to you, or see much less of that person?	

SECTION C—AFTER IDENTIFYING A POTENTIAL PROBLEM AREA, YOU MAY WANT TO ASK MORE SPECIFIC QUESTIONS ABOUT THE FOLLOWING:

Notes

C1	*Interpersonal Disputes*	
1.	What is (was) the disagreement or dispute about?	
2.	What do you see as your problems?	
3.	What are your wishes in the relationship?	
4.	What does _____ want in this relationship?	
5.	How has _____ disappointed you in this relationship?	
6.	How do you think you might have disappointed him/her?	
7.	Do you think you could bring about the changes you would like?	
8.	Do you think you could bring about the changes _____ would like?	

(cont.)

Notes

9.	What are the ways you resolve your differences?	
10.	How do you and _____ usually work on the differences you have?	
11.	What resources do you have to bring about change?	
C2	***Role Transition***	
1.	How did your life change with your move, divorce, starting work (or whatever change has occurred)?	
2.	How did you feel about the change?	
3.	What relationships, if any, have been lost as a result of this change?	
4.	What people, if any, take their place?	
5.	What was life like for you before the change?	
6.	What were the good things about being _____ (a student, an employee, married, etc.)?	
7.	What were the not so good things about _____?	
8.	What are the good things about your new situation?	
9.	What are the not so good things about your new situation?	

(cont.)

Notes

C3	*Grief*	
1.	Can you talk about _____ (the deceased) with others?	
2.	Were you feeling sad or blue after the death?	
3.	Did you have trouble sleeping?	
4.	Could you carry on as usual?	
5.	Were you beyond tears?	
6.	Did you avoid going to the funeral or visiting the grave?	
7.	Are you afraid of having the same illness as the person who died?	
8.	Were the deceased person's possessions left in place?	
9.	Did you preserve his/her possessions?	
10.	Were there people you could count on to help you when _____ died?	

(cont.)

SECTION D—CLOSING THE INTERVIEW

		Notes
D I	*Always ask the patient:*	
1.	Is there anything else that you think is important for me to know about your relationships with people or about the various roles you have had (e.g., student, partner, parent, grandparent) in the course of your life?	
2.	Which of the problems we have talked about, if any, do you think is most linked to your most recent depression (or mania)?	

Other comments/notes:

APPENDIX 6. Therapist Checklist for Initial IPSRT Sessions

___ Assess patient's current mood state, symptoms, and immediate medical needs.

___ Explain role of therapist (and of the psychiatrist, if different from the therapist).

___ Educate patient about medication.

    ___ Listen for and address patient's fears and concerns regarding medication.

    ___ Discuss side effects.

___ Instruct patient in the use of emergency procedures.

___ With the patient's permission, meet with significant other or family member to hear concerns and gather collateral information and history.

___ Introduce psychoeducation regarding bipolar disorder.

___ Review with patient his or her history of mood episodes using illness history timeline.

    ___ Identify antecedents and consequences.

    ___ Assess the impact of mood disturbances on the patient's life.

    ___ Assess the impact of any treatment (medication and/or therapy) the patient has had.

    ___ Appraise the impact of severe life events on mood episodes.

___ Conduct the interpersonal inventory.

    ___ Review with patient significant relationships, past and present.

    ___ Identify current problems in relationships.

___ Identify recurrent problems and themes in relationships.

___ Select interpersonal problem area with patient.

___ Educate patient about social rhythms and importance of circadian integrity.

___ Introduce the Social Rhythm Metric as a useful tool in promoting circadian integrity.

    ___ Train patient in use of the SRM.

___ Encourage patient to monitor and discuss relationship between affective instability and social rhythms.

Note: If the patient is acutely ill, symptom management may take priority over other therapeutic issues until the patient has stabilized.

From *Treating Bipolar Disorder: A Clinician's Guide to Interpersonal Social Rhythm Therapy* by Ellen Frank. Copyright 2005 by The Guilford Press. Permission to photocopy this appendix is granted to purchasers of this book for personal use only (see copyright page for details).

Week of _____

Activity	Target time						
	Mon	Tues	Wed	Thur	Fri	Sat	Sun
Out of bed							
First contact (in person or by phone) with another person							
Have morning beverage							
Have breakfast							
Go outside for the first time							
Start work, school, housework, volunteer activities, child or family care							
Have lunch							
Take an afternoon nap							
Have dinner							
Physical exercise							
Have an evening snack/drink							
Watch evening TV news program							
Watch another TV program							
Activity A							
Activity B							
Return home (last time)							
Go to bed							

From *Treating Bipolar Disorder: A Clinician's Guide to Interpersonal Social Rhythm Therapy* by Ellen Frank. Copyright 2005 by The Guilford Press. Permission to photocopy this appendix is granted to purchasers of this book for personal use only (see copyright page for details).

APPENDIX 8. Future Stabilization Goals Chart

Activity	Goal	Target date
_____	_____	_____
_____	_____	_____
_____	_____	_____
_____	_____	_____
_____	_____	_____
_____	_____	_____
_____	_____	_____
_____	_____	_____
_____	_____	_____
_____	_____	_____
_____	_____	_____
_____	_____	_____

Other person involvement	Goal	Target date
_____	_____	_____
_____	_____	_____
_____	_____	_____
_____	_____	_____
_____	_____	_____
_____	_____	_____
_____	_____	_____
_____	_____	_____
_____	_____	_____
_____	_____	_____
_____	_____	_____
_____	_____	_____

From *Treating Bipolar Disorder: A Clinician's Guide to Interpersonal Social Rhythm Therapy* by Ellen Frank. Copyright 2005 by The Guilford Press. Permission to photocopy this appendix is granted to purchasers of this book for personal use only (see copyright page for details).

APPENDIX 9. Resources

U.S. ORGANIZATIONS

The Depression and Bipolar Support Alliance (DBSA)
730 North Franklin Street, Suite 501
Chicago, IL 60610
Phone: (800) 826-3632
Website: www.dbsalliance.org

DBSA is the largest patient-run, illness-specific organization. Visit the website for free educational materials or call the toll-free line. There is information on resources available on depression, manic–depression, and related mood disorders.

National Mental Health Association (NMHA)
1021 Prince Street
Alexandria, VA 22314
Phone: (800) 969-6642
Website: www.nmha.org

This organization offers information on clinical depression and other mental health topics.

National Institute of Mental Health (NIMH)—Public Inquiries
6001 Executive Boulevard, Room 8184, MSC 9663
Bethesda, MD 20892-9663
Phone: (301) 443-4513
Fax: (301) 443-4279
Website: www.nimh.nih.gov

NIMH is part of the National Institutes of Health and offers a considerable amount of information on depression and other mental illnesses.

National Alliance for the Mentally Ill (NAMI)
Colonial Place Three
2107 Wilson Blvd., Suite 300
Arlington, VA 22201-3042
Phone: (703) 524-7600; 1-800-859-NAMI
Fax: (703) 5243-9094
Website: www.nami.org

NAMI is a nonprofit, grassroots, self-help support and advocacy organization of consumers, families, and friends of people with severe mental illnesses.

(cont.)

From *Treating Bipolar Disorder: A Clinician's Guide to Interpersonal Social Rhythm Therapy* by Ellen Frank. Copyright 2005 by The Guilford Press. Permission to photocopy this appendix is granted to purchasers of this book for personal use only (see copyright page for details).

Depression and Related Affective Disorders Association (DRADA)
2330 West Joppa Road, Suite 100
Lutherville, MD 21093
Phone: (410) 583-2919
Fax: (410) 583-2964
Website: www.drada.org

DRADA is a community organization that serves individuals affected by a depressive illness, family members, health care professionals, and the general public.

Lithium Information Center
Madison Institute of Medicine
7617 Mineral Point Road, Suite 300
Madison, WI 53717
Phone: (608) 827-2470
Fax: (608) 827-2479
Website: www.miminc.org

The Lithium Information Center at the Madison Institute of Medicine is a resource for information on lithium treatment of bipolar disorders and on other medical and biological applications of lithium.

FOREIGN ORGANIZATIONS*

GAMIAN (Global Alliance of Mental Illness Advocacy Networks) is a not-for-profit international organization with its headquarters in New York City. It is a nonpolitical and nonsectarian network of organizations and individuals concerned about mental health. Acting as a community, the members of GAMIAN are committed to the empowerment of consumers to seek appropriate professional health care treatment for mental illness without fear of social stigma and with the recognition that such appropriate treatment will improve the quality of life of patients, their families, and their communities. GAMIAN is committed to promoting awareness of the constantly evolving knowledge about the causes, consequences, and treatments of mental illness.

Brazil
ABRATA
http://www.ABRATA.com.br

Canada
Mood Disorders Society of Canada
www.mooddisorderscanada.ca

Denmark
Depressions Foreningen
www.depressionsforeningen.dk

Israel
Enosh
enosh.org.il

(cont.)

Resources *(page 3 of 3)*

Italy
Fondazione IDEA
www.fondazioneidea.it

Netherlands
Verenigingvoor Manisch–Depressieven en Betrokkenen
www.vmdb.nl

Scotland
Bipolar Fellowship Scotland
www.bipolarscotland.org.co.uk

Spain
A.B.D.V.
www.abdv.org

*Obtained from the GAMIAN website at www.gamian.org/default.asp.

Mood Disorder Monitoring Chart

		14																
		12																
		10																
Mania Score		8																
		6																
		4																
		2																
		0																
SRM Score																		
		0																
		2																
Depression Score		6																
		8																
		10																
		12																
		14																
Visit No.																		

From *Treating Bipolar Disorder: A Clinician's Guide to Interpersonal Social Rhythm Therapy* by Ellen Frank. Copyright 2005 by The Guilford Press. Permission to photocopy this appendix is granted to purchasers of this book for personal use only (see copyright page for details).

References

Altshuler, L., Suppes, T., Black, D., Nolen, W. A., Keck, P. E., Jr., Frye, M. A., et al. (2003). Impact of antidepressant discontinuation after acute bipolar depression remission on rates of depressive relapse at 1-year follow-up. *American Journal of Psychiatry, 160*(7), 1252, 1262.

American Psychiatric Association. (1994). *Diagnostic and statistical manual of mental disorders* (4th ed.). Washington, DC: Author.

American Psychiatric Association. (2000). *Diagnostic and statistical manual of mental disorders* (4th ed., text rev.). Washington, DC: Author.

American Psychiatric Association. (2002). Practice guidelines for the treatment of patients with bipolar disorder (Rev.). *American Journal of Psychiatry, 159*(4, April Suppl.).

Andrade, A. C. F., Frank, E., Neto, F. L., Lafer, B., & Moraes, C. T. L. (2004, June). *Interpersonal problems of bipolar patients: A cross-cultural assessment study.* Rapid communications session conducted at the First International Conference on Interpersonal Psychotherapy, Pittsburgh, PA.

Angus, L., & Gillies, L. A. (1994). Counseling the borderline client: an interpersonal approach. *Canadian Journal of Counselling/Revue Canadienne de Counselling, 28*, 69–82.

Aschoff, J. (1981). *Handbook of behavioral neurobiology: Vol. 4. Biological rhythms.* New York: Plenum Press.

Avery, D., Wildschiodtz, G., & Rafaelsen, O. J. (1982). REM latency and temperature in affective disorder before and after treatment. *Biological Psychiatry, 17*(4), 463–470.

Barden, N., Reul, J. M. H. M., & Holsboer, F. (1995). Do antidepressants stabilize mood through actions on the hypothalamic–pituitary–adrenocortical system? *Trends in Neurosciences, 18*(1), 6–11.

Basco, M. R., & Rush, A. J. (2005). *Cognitive-behavioral therapy for bipolar disorder* (2nd ed.). New York: Guilford Press.

Bauer, M. S., Callahan, A. M., Jampala, C., Petty, F., Sajatovic, M., Schaefer, V., et al. (1999). Clinical practice guidelines for bipolar disorder from the Department of Veterans Affairs. *Journal of Clinical Psychiatry, 60*, 9–21.

Bauer, M. S., & McBride, L. (1996). *Structured group psychotherapy for bipolar disorder: The Life Goals Program.* New York: Springer.

Bech, P., Bolwig, T. G., Kramp, P., & Rafaelsen, O. J. (1979). The Bech–Rafaelsen Mania Scale and the Hamilton Depression Scale. *Acta Psychiatrica Scandinavia, 59*, 420–430.

Beck, A. T. (1967). *Depression: Clinical, experimental, and theoretical aspects.* New York: Harper & Row.

Beck, A. T., Rush, A. J., Shaw, B. F., & Emery, G. (1979). *Cognitive therapy of depression*. New York: Guilford Press.

Beck, A. T., Steer, R. A., & Brown, G. K. (1996). *Beck Depression Inventory–II (BDI-II)*. San Antonio, TX: Psychological Corporation.

Beck, A. T., Ward, C. H., Mendelson, M., Mock, J., & Erbaugh, J. (1961). An inventory for measuring depression. *Archives of General Psychiatry, 4*, 561–571.

Bertelsen, A. B., Harvald, A. B., & Hauge, H. (1977). A Danish twin study of manic–depressive disorders. *British Journal of Psychiatry, 130*, 330–351.

Birmaher, B. (2004). *New hope for children with bipolar disorder*. New York: Three Rivers Press.

Bowden, C. L., Calabrese, J. R., Sachs, G., Yatham, L. N., Asghar, S. A., Hompland, M., et al. (2003). A placebo-controlled 18-month trial of lamotrigine and lithium maintenance treatment in recently manic or hypomanic patients with bipolar I disorder. *Archives of General Psychiatry, 60*, 392–400.

Brown, G. B., & Harris, T. (1979). *The social origins of depression*. London: Tavistock.

Brown, G. W., Birley, J. L. T., & Wing, J. K. (1972). Influence of family life on the course of schizophrenic disorders: A replication. *British Journal of Psychiatry, 121*, 241–258.

Calabrese, J. R., Bowden, C. L., Sachs, G. S., Ascher, J. A., Monaghan, E., & Rudd, G. D. (1999). A double-blind placebo-controlled study of lamotrigine monotherapy in outpatients with bipolar I depression. *Journal of Clinical Psychiatry, 60*, 79–88.

Calabrese, J. R., Bowden, C. L., Sachs, G., Yatham, L. N., Behnke, K., Mehtonen, O. P., et al. (2003). A placebo-controlled 18-month trial of lamotrigine and lithium maintenance treatment in recently depressed patients with bipolar I disorder. *Journal of Clinical Psychiatry, 64*, 1013–1024.

Cartwright, R. D. (1983). Rapid eye movement sleep characteristics during and after mood-disturbing events. *Archives of General Psychiatry, 40*, 197–201.

Cassano, G. B., Banti, S., Mauri, M., Dell'Osso, L., Miniati, M., Maser, J. D., et al. (1999b). Internal consistency and discriminant validity of the Structured Clinical Interview for Panic–Agoraphobic Spectrum (SCI-PAS). *International Journal of Methods in Psychiatric Research, 8*, 138–145.

Cassano, G. B., Dell'Osso, L., Frank, E., Miniati, M., Fagiolini, A., Shear, K., et al. (1999a). The bipolar spectrum: A clinical reality in search of diagnostic criteria and an assessment methodology. *Journal of Affective Disorders, 54*, 319–328.

Cassano, G. B., Frank, E., Miniati, M., Rucci, P., Fagiolini, A., Pini, S., et al. (2002). Conceptual underpinnings and empirical support for mood spectrum. *Psychiatric Clinics of North America, 25*, 699–712.

Cassano, G. B., Michelini, S., Shear, M. K., Coli, E., Maser, J. D., & Frank, E. (1997). The panic–agoraphobic spectrum: A descriptive approach to the assessment and treatment of subtle symptoms. *American Journal of Psychiatry, 154*(Special Suppl.), 27–38.

Cassidy, F., Ritchie, J. C., & Carroll, B. J. (1998). Plasma dexamethasone concentration and cortisol response during manic episodes. *Biological Psychiatry, 43*(10), 747–754.

Cerbone, M. J., Mayo, J. A., Cuthbertson, B. A., & O'Connell, R. A. (1992). Group therapy as an adjunct to medication in the management of affective disorder. *Group, 16*, 174–187.

Cervantes, P., Gelber, S., Kin, F. N., Nair, N. P., & Schwartz, G. (2001). Circadian secretion of cortisol in bipolar disorder. *Journal of Psychiatry and Neuroscience, 26*(5), 411–416.

Clarkin, J. F., Carpenter, D., Hull, J., Wilner, P., & Glick, I. (1998). Effects of psychoeducational intervention for married patients with bipolar disorder and their spouses. *Psychiatric Services, 49*, 531–533.

Clarkin, J. F., Glick, I. D., Haas, G. L., Spencer, J. H., Lewis, A. B., Peyser, J., et al. (1990). A randomized clinical trial of inpatient family intervention: V. Results for affective disorders. *Journal of Affective Disorders, 18*, 17–28.

Clarkin, J. F., Haas, G. L., & Glick, I. D. (Eds.). (1988). *Affective disorders and the family: Assessment and treatment*. New York: Guilford Pres.

Colom, F., Vieta, E., Martinez-Aran, A., Reinares, M., Goikolea, J. M., Benabarre, A., et al. (2003).

A randomized trial on the efficacy of group psychoeducation in the prophylaxis of recur-rences in bipolar patients whose disease is in remission. *Archives of General Psychiatry, 60*(4), 402–407.

Coryell, W., Scheftner, W., Keller, M., Endicott, J., Mase, J., & Klerman, G. L. (1993). The enduring psychosocial consequences of mania and depression. *American Journal of Psychiatry, 150,* 720–727.

Craighead, W. E., Miklowitz, D. J., Vajk, F. C., & Frank, E. (1998). Psychosocial treatments for bi-polar disorder. In P. E. Nathan, & J. M. Gorman (Eds.), *A guide to treatments that work* (pp. 240–248). New York: Oxford University Press.

Crits-Cristoph, P., Frank, E., Chambless, D. C., Brody, C., & Karp, J. (1995). Training in empirically validated treatments: What are clinical psychology students learning? *Professional Psychol-ogy: Research and Practice, 26*(5), 514–522.

Cutler, N. R., & Post, R. M. (1982). Life course of illness in untreated manic–depressive patients. *Comprehensive Psychiatry, 23,* 101–115.

Davenport, Y. B., Ebert, M. H., Adland, M. L., & Goodwin, F. K. (1977). Couples group therapy as an adjunct to lithium maintenance of the manic patient. *American Journal of Orthopsychiatry, 47,* 495–502.

Ehlers, C. L., Frank, E., & Kupfer, D. J. (1988). Social *zeitgebers* and biological rythms. A unified approach to understanding the etiology of depression. *Archives of General Psychiatry, 45*(10), 948–952.

Ehlers, C. L., Kupfer, D. J., Frank, E., & Monk, T. H.(1993). Biological rhythms and depression: The role of *zeitgebers* and *zeitstorers. Depression, 1,* 285–293.

Ehlers, C. L., Wall, T. L., Wyss, S. P., & Chaplin, R. I. (1988). A peer separation model of depres-sion in rats. In G. F. Koob, C. L. Ehlers, & D. J. Kupfer (Eds.), *Animal models of depression* (pp. 99–110). Boston: Birhauser.

Ellicott, A., Hammen, C., Gitlin, M., Brown, G., & Jamison, K. (1990). Life events and the course of bipolar disorder. *American Journal of Psychiatry, 147,* 1194–1198.

Fagiolini, A., Dell'Osso, L., Pini, S., Armani, A., Bouanani, S., Rucci, P., et al. (1999). Validity and reliability of a new instrument for assessing mood symptomatology: The structured clinical interview for mood spectrum (SCI-MOODS). *International Journal of Methods in Psychiatric Research, 8,* 71–82.

Fagiolini, A., Kupfer, D. J., Houck, P., Novick, D. M., & Frank, E. (2003). Obesity as a correlate of outcome in patients with bipolar I disorder. *American Journal of Psychiatry, 160,* 112–117.

Falloon, I. R. H., Boyd, J. L., McGill, C. W., Williamson, W., Razoni, J., Moss, H. B., et al. (1985). Family management in the prevention of morbidity of schizophrenia. *Archives of General Psychiatry, 42,* 887–896.

Fieve, R. (1975). The lithium clinic: A new model for the delivery of psychiatric services. *American Journal of Psychiatry, 132*(10), 1018–1022.

First, M. B., Spitzer, R. L., Gibbon, M., & Williams, J. B. W. (2002). *Structured Clinical Interview for DSM-IV-TR Axis I Disorders, Research Version, Patient Edition (SCID-I/P).* New York: Bio-metrics Research, New York State Psychiatric Institute.

Frances, A. J., Kahn, D. A., Carpenter, D., Docherty, J. P., & Donovan, S. L. (1998). The expert con-sensus guidelines for treating depression in bipolar disorder. *Journal of Clinical Psychiatry, 59*(Suppl. 4), 73–79.

Frank, E., Cyranowski, J. M., Rucci, P., Shear, M. K., Fagiolini, A., Thase, M. E., et al. (2002). Clini-cal significance of lifetime panic spectrum symptoms in the treatment of patients with bipo-lar I disorder. *Archives of General Psychiatry, 59,* 905–912.

Gelenberg, A. J., Kane, J. M., Keller, M. B., Labori, P., Rosenbaum, J. F., Cole, K., & Lavelle, J. (1989). Comparison of standard and low serum levels of lithium for maintenance treatment of bipolar disorder. *New England Journal of Medicine, 321,* 1489–1493.

Gershon, E. S., Hamovit, J., Guroff, J. J., Dibble, E., Leckman, J. F., Sceery, W., et al. (1982). A fam-ily study of schizoaffective, bipolar I, bipolar II, unipolar, and normal control probands. *Ar-chives of General Psychiatry, 39,* 1157–1167.

Gershon, S., & Yuwiler, A. A. (1960). A specific pharmacological approach to the treatment of mania. *Journal of Neuropsychiatry, 1*, 229–241.

Gillin, J. C., Buchsbaum, M., Wu, J., Clark, C., & Bunney, W. (2001). Sleep deprivation as a model experimental antidepressant treatment: Findings from functional brain imaging. *Depression and Anxiety, 14*(1), 37–49.

Gitlin, M. J., Swendsen, J., Heller, T. L., & Hammen, C. (1995). Relapse and impairment in bipolar disorder. *American Journal of Psychiatry, 152*, 1635–1640.

Glick, I. D., Clarkin, J. F., Haas, G. L., Spencer, J. H., & Chen, C. L. (1991). A randomized clinical trial of inpatient family intervention: VI. Mediating variables and outcome. *Family Process, 30*, 85–99.

Goetze, U., & Toelle, R. (1987). Circadian rhythm of free urinary cortisol, temperature and heart rate in endogenous depressives and under antidepressant therapy. *Neuropsychobiology, 18*(4), 175–184.

Golden, R. N., Heine, A. D., Ekstrom, R. D., Bebchuk, J. M., Leatherman, M. E., & Garbutt, J. C. (2002). A longitudinal study of serotonergic function in depression. *Neuropsychopharmacology, 26*(5), 653–659.

Goodwin, F. K., & Jamison, K. R. (1990). *Manic–depressive illness.* New York: Oxford University Press.

Goodwin, G. M. (2003). Evidence-based guidelines for treating bipolar disorder: Recommendations from the British Association for Psychopharmacology. *Journal of Psychopharmacology, 17*, 149–173.

Gordon, N. P., Cleary, P. D., Parlan, C. E., & Czeisler, C. A. (1986). The prevalence and health impact of shiftwork. *American Journal of Public Health, 76*, 1225–1228.

Graves, J. S. (1993). Living with mania: A study of outpatient group psychotherapy for bipolar patients. *American Journal of Psychotherapy, 47*, 113–126.

Haas, G. L., Glick, I. D., Clarkin, J. F., Spencer, J. H., Lewis, A. B., Peyser, J., et al. (1988). Inpatient family intervention: A randomized clinical trial: II. Results at hospital discharge. *Archives of General Psychiatry, 45*, 217–224.

Halbreich, U., & Montgomery, S. A. (Eds.). (2000). *Pharmacotherapy for mood, anxiety, and cognitive disorders.* Washington, DC: American Psychiatric Press.

Hamilton, M. (1960). A rating scale for depression. *Journal of Neurology, Neurosurgery and Psychiatry, 23*, 56–62.

Hardman, J. G., Limbird, L. E., & Goodman Gilman, A. (Eds.). (2001). *Goodman and Gilman's pharmacological basis of therapeutics* (10th ed.). New York: McGraw-Hill.

Harrow, M., Goldberg, J. F., Grossman, L. S., & Meltzer, H. Y. (1990). Outcome in manic disorders: A naturalistic follow-up study. *Archives of General Psychiatry, 47*, 665–671.

Heckers, S., Stone, D., Walsh, J., Shick, J., Koul, P., & Benes, F. M. (2002). Differential hippocampal expression of glutamic acid decarboxylase 65 and 67 messenger RNA in bipolar disorder and schizophrenia. *Archives of General Psychiatry, 59*, 521–529.

Himmelhoch, J. M., Thase M. E., Mallinger, A. G., & Houck, P. R. (1991). Tranylcypromine versus imipramine in anergic bipolar depression. *American Journal of Psychiatry, 148*, 910–916.

Hlastala, S. A., & Frank, E. (2000). Biology versus environment: Stressors in the pathophysiology of bipolar disorder. In J. Soares & S. Gershon (Eds.), *Bipolar disorders: Basic mechanisms and therapeutic implications* (pp. 353–372). New York: Dekker.

Hlastala, S. A., Frank, E., Kowalski, J., Sherrill, J. T., Tu, X. M., Anderson, B., & Kupfer, D. J. (2000). Stressful life events, bipolar disorder, and the "Kindling Model." *Journal of Abnormal Psychology, 109*, 777–786.

Hlastala, S. A., Frank, E., Mallinger, A. G., Thase, M. E., Ritenour, A. M., & Kupfer, D. J. (1997). Bipolar depression: An underestimated treatment challenge. *Depression, 5*, 73–83.

Hofer, M. A. (1984). Relationships as regulators: A psychobiologic perspective on bereavement. *Psychosomatic Medicine, 46*, 183–197.

Hogarty, E. G., Anderson, C. M., Reiss, D. J., Kornblith, S. J., Greenwald, D. P., Javna, C. D., & Madonia, J. J. (1986). Family psychoeducation, social skills training, and maintenance chemotherapy in the aftercare treatment of schizophrenia: I. One-year effects of a controlled study on relapse and expressed emotion. *Archives of General Psychiatry, 43,* 633–642.

Holsboer, F. (1995). Neuroendocrinology of mood disorders. In F. E. Bloom, & D. J. Kupfer (Eds.), *Psychopharmacology: The fourth generation of progress: An official publication of the American College of Neuropsychopharmacology* (pp. 957–970). New York: Raven Press.

Holsboer, F. (2000). Current theories on the pathophysiology of mood disorders. In U. Halbreich & S. A. Montgomery (Eds.), *Pharmacotherapy for mood, anxiety, and cognitive disorders* (pp. 13–36). Washington, DC: American Psychiatric Press.

Honig, A., Hofman, A., Rozendaal, N., & Dingemanns, P. (1997). Psychoeducation in bipolar disorder: Effect on expressed emotion. *Psychiatry Research, 72,* 17–22.

Jacobs, L. I. (1982). Cognitive therapy of postmanic and postdepressive dysphoria in bipolar illness. *American Journal of Psychotherapy, 36,* 450–458.

Jacobson, N. S., Dobson, K. S., Truax, P. A., Addis, M. E., Koerner, K., Gollan, J. K., et al. (1996). A component analysis of cognitive-behavioral treatment for depression. *Journal of Consulting and Clinical Psychology, 64,* 295–304.

James, S. P., Weh, T. A., Sack, D. A., Parry, B. L., & Rosenthal, N. E. (1985). Treatment of seasonal affective disorder with light in the evening. *British Journal of Psychiatry, 147,* 424–428.

Janowsky, D. S., & Overstreet, D. H. (1995) The role of acetylcholine mechanisms in mood disorders. In F. E. Bloom & D. J. Kupfer (Eds.), *Psychopharmacology: The fourth generation of progress: An official publication of the American College of Neuropsychopharmacology* (pp. 945–956). New York: Raven Press.

Jauhar, P., & Weller, M. P. L. (1982). Psychiatric morbidity and time zone changes: A study of patients from Heathrow Airport. *British Journal of Psychiatry, 140,* 231–235.

Judd, L. L., Akiskal, H. S., Schettler, P. J., Endicott, J., Maser, J., Solomon, D. A., et al. (2002). The long-term natural history of the weekly symptomatic status of bipolar I disorder. *Archives of General Psychiatry, 59,* 530–537.

Ketter, T., Tohen, M., Vieta, E., Calabrese, J., Andersen, S., Detke, H. C., et al. (2003, May). Open-label maintenance treatment for bipolar depression using olanzapine or olanzapine/fluoxetine combination. Poster session presented at the 43rd annual meeting of the New Clinical Drug Evaluation Unit, Boca Raton, FL.

Klein, K. E., & Wegmann, H. M. (1974). *The resynchronization of human circadian rhythms after transmeridian flights as a result of flight direction and mode of activity.* Tokyo: Igaku Shoin.

Klerman, G. L., Weissman, M. M., Rounsaville, B. J., & Chevron, E. S. (Eds.). (1984). *Interpersonal psychotherapy of depression.* New York: Basic Books.

Knutsson, A., Akerstedt, T., Jonsson, B. G., & Orth-Gomer, K. (1986). Increased risk of ischemic heart disease in shift workers. *Lancet, 2,* 89–92.

Kripke, D. F., & Robinson, D. (1985). Ten years with a lithium group. *McLean Hospital Journal, 10,* 1–11.

Kupfer, D. J. (1978). Application of EEG sleep for the differential diagnosis and treatment of affective disorders. *Pharmacopsychiatry, Neurology, and Psychopharmacology, 11,* 17–26.

Kupfer, D. J., Frank, E., Grochocinski, V. J., Cluss, P. A., Houck, P. R., & Stapf, D. A. (2002). Demographic and clinical characteristics of individuals in a bipolar disorder case registry. *Journal of Clinical Psychiatry, 63,* 120–125.

Kupfer, D. J., Frank, E., Grochocinski, V. J., Luther, J. F., Houck, P. R., Swartz, H. A., & Mallinger, A. G. (2000). Stabilization in the treatment of mania, depression and mixed states. *Acta Neuropsychiatrica, 12,* 110–114.

Kupfer, D. J., Reynolds, C., Weiss, B. L., & Foster, F. G. (1974). Lithium carbonate and sleep in affective disorders: Further considerations. *Archives of General Psychiatry, 30,* 79–84.

Kusumaker, V., Yatham, L. N., Haslam, D. R. S., Parikh, S. V., Matte, R., Sharma, V., et al. (1997). The foundations of effective management of bipolar disorder. *Canadian Journal of Psychiatry, 42*(Suppl. 2), 69S–73S.

Lam, D. H., Jones, S. H., Hayward, P., & Bright, J. A. (1999). *Cognitive therapy for bipolar disorder.* Chichester: Wiley.

Lam, D. H., Watkins, E. R., Hayward, P., Bright, J., Wright, K., Kerr, N., et al. (2002). A randomized controlled study of cognitive therapy for relapse prevention for bipolar affective disorder: Outcome of the first year. *Archives of General Psychiatry, 60*(2), 145–152.

Leatherman, M. E., Ekstrom, R. D., Corrigan, M., Carson, S. W., Mason, G., & Golden, R. N. (1993). Central serotonergic changes following antidepressant treatment: A neuroendocrine assessment. *Psychopharmacology Bulletin, 29*(2), 149–154.

Lewy, A. J. (1995). Circadian phase sleep and mood disorders. In F. E. Bloom & D. J. Kupfer (Eds.), *Psychopharmacology: The fourth generation of progress: An official publication of the American College of Neuropsychopharmacology* (pp. 1879–1894). New York: Raven Press.

Lewy, A. J., Sack, R. L., & Singer, C. M. (1985). Treating phase typed chronobiological sleep and mood disorders using appropriately timed bright artificial light. *Psychopharmacology Bulletin, 21*, 368–372.

Maes, M., & Meltzer, H. Y. (1995). The serotonin hypothesis of major depression. In F. E. Bloom & D. J. Kupfer (Eds.), *Psychopharmacology: The fourth generation of progress: An official publication of the American College of Neuropsychopharmacology* (pp. 933–944). New York: Raven Press.

Maj, M., Pirozzi, R., & Kemali, D. (1989). Long-term outcome of lithium prophylaxis in patients initially classified as complete responders. *Psychopharmacology, 98*, 535–538.

Malkoff-Schwartz, S., Frank, E., Anderson, B., Sherrill, J. T., Siegel, L., Patterson, D., & Kupfer, D. J. (1998). Stressful life events and social rhythm disruption in the onset of manic and depressive bipolar episodes: A preliminary investigation. *Archives of General Psychiatry, 55*, 702–707.

Manji, H. K., Drevets, W. C., & Charney, D. S. (2001). The cellular neurobiology of depression. *Nature Medicine, 7*, 541–547.

Manji, H. K., & Lenox, R. H. (1999). Protein kinase C signaling in the brain: Molecular transduction of mood stabilization in the treatment of manic–depressive illness. *Biological Psychiatry, 46*(10), 1328–1351.

Markar, H. R., & Mander, A. J. (1989). Efficacy of lithium prophylaxis in clinical practice. *British Journal of Psychiatry, 155*, 496–500.

Markowitz, J. C., Skodol, A. E., & Blieberg, K. (in press). Interpersonal psychotherapy for borderline disorder: Possible mechanisms of change. *Journal of Clinical Psychiatry.*

Mauri, M., Borri, C., Baldassari, S., Benvenuti, A., Cassano, G. B., Rucci, P., et al. (2000). Acceptability and psychometric properties of the Structured Clinical Interview for Anorexic-Bulimic Spectrum (SCI-ABS). *International Journal of Methods in Psychiatric Research, 9*, 68–78.

Mendelson, W. B., James, S. P., Rosenthal, N. E., Sack, D. A., Wehr, T. A., Garnett, D., & Weingartne, H. (1986). The experience of insomnia. In C. Shagass, R. C. Josiassen, W. H. Bridger, K. J. Weiss, D. Stoff, & G. M. Simpson (Eds.), *Biological Psychiatry 1985: Proceedings of the 4th World Congress of Biological Psychiatry* (pp. 1005–1006). New York: Elsevier.

Mendelwicz, J., Linkowski, P., Kerkhofs, M., Desmedt, D., Goldstein, J., Copinschi, G., & Van Cauter, E. (1985). Diurnal hypersecretion of growth hormone in depression. *Journal of Clinical Endocrinology and Metabolism, 60*, 505–512.

Miklowitz, D. J., & Goldstein, M. J. (1990). Behavioral family treatment for patients with bipolar affective disorder [Special issue]. Recent developments in the behavioral treatment of chronic psychiatric illness. *Behavior Modification, 14*, 457–489.

Miklowitz, D. J., & Goldstein, M. J. (1997). *Bipolar disorder: A family-focused treatment approach.* New York: Guilford Press.

Miklowitz, D. J., Goldstein, M. J., Neuchterlein, K. H., Snyder, K. S., & Mintz, J. (1988). Family factors and the course of bipolar affective disorder. *Archives of General Psychiatry, 45*, 225–231.

Miklowitz, D. J., Richards, J. A., George, E. L., Frank, E., Suddath, R. L., Powell, K. B., & Sacher, J. A. (2003). Integrated family and individual therapy for bipolar disorder: Results of a treatment development study. *Journal of Clinical Psychiatry, 64*, 182–191.

Miklowitz, D. J., Simoneau, T. L., George, E. L., Richards, J. A., Kalbag, A., Sachs-Ericsson, N., & Suddath, R. (2000). Family-focused treatment of bipolar disorder: 1-year effects of a psychoeducational program in conjunction with pharmacotherapy. *Biological Psychiatry, 48*(6), 582–592.

Modell, S., Ising, M., Holsboer, F., & Lauer, C. (2002). The Munich vulnerability study on affective disorders: Stability of polysomnographic findings over time. *Biological Psychiatry, 52*(5), 430.

Monk, T. H. (1988). Coping with the stress of shiftwork. *Work Stress, 2,* 169–172.

Monk, T. H., Flaherty, J. F., Frank, E., Hoskinson, K., & Kupfer, D. J. (1990). The social rhythm metric: An instrument to quantify the daily rhythms of life. *Journal of Nervous and Mental Disorders, 178,* 120–126.

Monk, T. H., Frank, E., Potts, J. M., & Kupfer, D. J. (2002). A simple way to measure daily lifestyle regularity. *Journal of Sleep Research, 11*(3), 183–190.

Monk, T. H., Kupfer, D. J., Frank, E., & Ritenour, A. M. (1991). The social rhythm metric (SRM): Measuring daily social rhythms over 12 weeks. *Psychiatry Research, 36,* 195–207.

Monk, T. H., Reynolds, C. F., III, Machen, M. A., & Kupfer, D. J. (1992). Daily social rhythms in the elderly and their relation to objectively recorded sleep. *Sleep, 15,* 322–329.

Montgomery, A. (1979). A new depression scale designed to be sensitive to change. *British Journal of Psychiatry, 134,* 382–389.

Newman, C. F., Leahy, R. L., Beck, A. T., Reilly-Harrington, N. A., & Gyulai, L. (2001). *Bipolar disorder: A cognitive therapy approach.* Washington, DC: American Psychological Association.

Nofzinger, E. A., & Keshavan, M. (1995). Sleep disturbances associated with neuropsychiatric disease. In F. E. Bloom & D. J. Kupfer (Eds.), *Psychopharmacology: The fourth generation of progress: An official publication of the American College of Neuropsychopharmacology* (pp. 1945–1960). New York: Raven Press.

O'Connell, R. A., Mayo, J. A., Flatow, L., Cuthbertson, B., & O'Brien, B. E. (1991). Outcome of bipolar disorder on long-term treatment with lithium. *British Journal of Psychiatry, 159,* 132–129.

Otto, M. W., Reilly-Harrington, N. A., & Sachs, G. S. (2003). Psychoeducational and cognitive-behavioral strategies in the management of bipolar disorder. *Journal of Affective Disorders, 73,* 171–181.

Palmer, A. G., Williams, H., & Adams, M. (1995). CBT in group format for bipolar affective disorder. *Behavioural and Cognitive Psychotherapy, 23,* 153–168.

Paykel, E. S., & Tanner, J. (1976). Live events, depressive relapse and maintenance treatment. *Psychological Medicine, 6,* 481–485.

Peet, M., & Harvey, N. S. (1991). Lithium maintenance: 1. A standard education programme for patients. *British Journal of Psychiatry, 158,* 197–200.

Perry, A., Tarrier, N., Morriss, R., McCarthy, E., & Limb, K. (1999). Randomized controlled trial of efficacy of teaching patients with bipolar disorder to identify early symptoms of relapse and obtain treatment. *British Medical Journal, 318,* 149–153.

Plotsky, P. M., Owens, M. J., & Nemeroff, C. B. (1995). Neuropeptide alterations in mood disorders. In F. E. Bloom & D. J. Kupfer (Eds.), *Psychopharmacology: The fourth generation of progress: An official publication of the American College of Neuropsychopharmacology* (pp. 971–982). New York: Raven Press.

Post, R. M., Jimerson, D. C., Ballenger, J. C., Lake, C. R., Uhde, T. W., & Goodwin, F. K. (1984). Cerebrospinal fluid norepinephrine and its metabolites in manic–depressive illness. In R. M. Post & J. C. Ballenger (Eds.), *Neurobiology of mood disorders: Vol 1. Frontiers of clinical neuroscience* (pp. 539–553). Baltimore: Williams & Wilkins.

Potter, W. Z., & Prien, R. F. (1989). *Report on the NIMH Workshop on the Treatment of Bipolar Disorder.* Unpublished manuscript, available from R. F. Prien, National Institute of Mental Health, Parklawn Building, 5600 Fishers Lane, Rockville, MD 20857.

Priebe, S., Wildgrube, C., & Muller-Oerlinghausen, B. (1989). Lithium prophylaxis and expressed emotion. *British Journal of Psychiatry, 154,* 396–399.

Rea, M. M., Tompson, M., Miklowitz, D. J., Goldstein, M. J., Hwang, S., & Mintz, J. (2003). Family-focused treatment vs. individual treatment for bipolar disorder: Results of a randomized clinical trial. *Journal of Consulting and Clinical Psychology, 71*(3), 482–92.

Regestein, Q. R., & Monk, T. H. (1991). Is the poor sleep of shift workers a disorder? *American Journal of Psychiatry, 148*, 1487–1493.

Riemann, D., Voderholzer, U., & Berger, M. (2002). Sleep and sleep–wake manipulations in bipolar depression. *Neuropsychobiology, 45*(Suppl. 1), 7–12.

Risch, S. C., Janowsky, D. S., Parker, D., Kalin, N. H., Aloi, J., Cohen, R. M., et al. (1984). Neuroendocrine abnormalities in affective disorders: Possible cholinergic mechanisms. In R. M. Post & J. C. Ballenger (Eds.), *Neurobiology of mood disorders: Vol 1. Frontiers of clinical neuroscience* (pp. 664–672). Baltimore: Williams & Wilkins.

Rush, A. J., Carmody, T., & Reimitz, P. E. (2000). The Inventory of Depressive Symptomatology (IDS): Clinician (IDS-C) and self-report (IDS-SR) ratings of depressive symptoms. *International Journal of Methods in Psychiatric Research, 9*, 45–59.

Rush, A. J., Giles, D. E., Schlesser, M. A., Fulton, C. L., Weissenburger, J. E., & Burns, C. T. (1986). The Inventory for Depressive Symptomatology (IDS): Preliminary findings. *Psychiatry Research, 18*, 65–87.

Rush, A. J., Giles, D. E., Schlesser, M. A., Orsulak, P. J., Parker, C. R., Jr., Weissenburger, J. E., et al. (1996). The dexamethasone suppression test in patients with mood disorders. *Journal of Clinical Psychiatry, 57*(10), 470–484.

Rush, A. J., Trivedi, M. H., Ibrahim, H. M., Carmody, T. J., Arnow, B., Klein, C. N., et al. (2003). The 16-item Quick Inventory of Depressive Symptomatology (QIDS), Clinician Rating (QIDS-C), and Self-Report (QIDS, SR): a psychometric evaluation in patients with chronic major depression. *Biological Psychiatry, 54*(5), 573–583.

Rutenfranz, J., Colquhoun, W. P., Knauth, P., & Ghata, J. N. (1977). Biomedical and psychosocial aspects of shift work: A review. *Scandinavian Journal of Work, Environment and Health, 3*, 165–182.

Rybakowski, J. K., & Twardowska, K. (1999). The dexamethasone/corticotropin-releasing hormone test in depression in bipolar and unipolar affective illness. *Journal of Psychiatric Research, 33*(5), 363–370.

Sack, D. A., Rosenthal, N. E., Parry, B. L, & Wehr, T. A. (1987). Biological rhythms in psychiatry. In H. Y. Meltzer (Ed.), *Psychopharmacology: The third generation of progress* (pp. 669–685). New York: Raven Press.

Schatzberg, A. F., & Schildkraut, J. J. (1995). Recent studies on norepinephrine systems in mood disorders. In F. E. Bloom & D. J. Kupfer (Eds.), *Psychopharmacology: The fourth generation of progress: An official publication of the American College of Neuropsychopharmacology* (pp. 911–920). New York: Raven Press.

Schou, M., Juel-Nielsen, N., Stromgren, E., & Voldby, H. (1954). The treatment of manic psychoses by the administration of lithium salts. *Journal of Neurology, Neurosurgery, and Psychiatry, 17*, 250–260.

Scott, J., Garland, A., & Moorhead, S. (2001). A pilot study of cognitive therapy in bipolar disorders. *Psychological Medicine, 31*(3), 459–67.

Sharma, V., Mazmanian, D. S., Persad, E., & Kueneman, K. M. (1997). Treatment of bipolar depression: A survey of Canadian psychiatrists. *Canadian Journal of Psychiatry, 42*, 298–302.

Shear, M. K., Cassano, G. B., Frank, E., Rucci, P., Rotondo, A., & Fagiolini, A. (2002). The panic-agoraphobic spectrum: Development, description, and clinical significance. *Psychiatric Clinics of North America, 25*, 739–756.

Shear, M. K., Greeno, C., Kang, J., Ludewig, D., Frank, E., Swartz, H. A., & Hanekamp, M. (2000). Diagnosis of non-psychotic patients in community clinics. *American Journal of Psychiatry, 157*, 581–587.

Sheehan, D. V., Lecrubier, Y., Sheehan, K. H., Amorim, P., Janavs, J., Weiller, E., et al. (1998). The Mini-International Neuropsychiatric Interview (M.I.N.I.): The development and validation of a structured diagnostic psychiatric interview for DSM-IV and ICD-10. *Journal of Clinical Psychiatry, 59*(Suppl. 20), 22–33.

Siever, L. J., Guttmacher, L. B., & Murphy, D. L. (1984). Serotonergic receptors: Evaluation of their possible role in the affective disorders. In R. M. Post & J. C. Ballenger (Eds.), *Neurobiology of mood disorders: Vol. 1. Frontiers of clinical neuroscience* (pp. 587–600). Baltimore: Williams & Wilkins.

Simon, G. E., Ludman, E. J., Unutzer, J., & Bauer, M. S. (2002). Design and implementation of a randomized trial evaluating systematic care for bipolar disorder. *Bipolar Disorders, 4*(4), 226–236.

Simon, G. E., Ludman, E. J., Unutzer, J., Bauer, M. S., Operskalski, B., & Rutter, C. (2005). Randomized trial of a population-based care program for people with bipolar disorder. *Psychological Medicine, 35*, 13–24.

Soldatos, C. R., & Bergiannaki, J. D. (2000). Sleep in depression and the effects of antidepressants on sleep. In U. Halbreich & S. A. Montgomery (Eds.), *Pharmacotherapy for mood, anxiety, and cognitive disorders* (pp. 255–272). Washington, DC: American Psychiatric Press.

Spencer, J. H., Glick, I. D., Haas, G. L., Clarkin, J. F., Lewis, A. B., Peyser, J., et al. (1988). A randomized clinical trial of inpatient family intervention: III. Effects at 6-month and 18-month follow-ups. *American Journal of Psychiatry, 145*, 1115–1121.

Suppes, T., Dennehy, A. C., Swan, C. L., Bowden, J. R., Calabrese, J. R., Hirschfeld, R. M. A., et al. (2002). Report of the Texas Consensus Conference Panel on medication treatment for bipolar disorder 2000. *Journal of Clinical Psychiatry, 63*, 288–299.

Suppes, T., Swann, A. C., Dennehy, E. B., Habermacher, E. D., Mason, M., Crismon, M. L., et al. (2001). Texas Medication Algorithm Project: Development and feasibility testing of a treatment algorithm for patients with bipolar disorder. *Journal of Clinical Psychiatry, 62*(6), 439–447.

Swartz, H. A., & Frank, E. (2001). Psychotherapy for bipolar depression: A phase-specific strategy? *Bipolar Disorders, 3*, 11–22.

Swartz, H. A., Frank, E., Shear, M. K., Thase, M. E., Fleming, M. A. D., & Scott, A. M. (2004). A pilot study of brief interpersonal psychotherapy for depression among women. *Psychiatric Services, 55*, 448–450.

Swartz, H. A., Pilkonis, P. A., Frank, E., Mallinger, A. G., Cherry, C. R., & Kupfer, D. J. (2000, January). *Bipolar disorder and comorbid borderline personality disorder: Treatment course and pharmacotherapy.* Poster session at the *Bipolar Disorder: From Pre-clinical to Clinical, Facing the New Millenium* meeting, Phoenix, AZ.

Swartz, H. A., Pilkonis, P. A., Frank, E., Proietti, J. M., & Scott, J. (2005). Acute treatment outcomes in patients with bipolar I disorder and co-morbid borderline personality disorder receiving medication and psychotherapy. *Bipolar Disorders, 7*, 192–197.

Szuba, M. P., Yager, A., Guze, B. H., Allen, E. M., & Baxter, Jr., L. R. (1992). Disruption of social circadian rhythms in major depression: A preliminary report. *Psychiatry Research, 42*, 221–230.

Tepas, D. I., & Monk, T. H. (1987). Work schedules. In G. Salvendy (Ed.), *Handbook of human factors* (pp. 819–843). New York: Wiley.

Thase, M. E., Frank, E., & Kupfer, D. J. (1985). Biological processes in major depression. In E. E. Beckham & W. R. Leber (Eds.), *Handbook of depression: Treatment, assessment, and research* (pp. 816–913). Homewood, IL: Dorsey Press.

Thase, M. E., Frank, E., Mallinger, A. G., Hamer, T., & Kupfer, D. J. (1992). Treatment of imipramine-resistant recurrent depression: III. Efficacy of monoamine oxidase inhibitors. *Journal of Clinical Psychiatry, 53*(1), 5–11.

Thase, M. E., Mallinger, A. G., McKnight, D., & Himmelhoch, J. M. (1992). Treatment of imipramine-resistant recurrent depression: IV. A double-blind crossover study of tranylcypromine for anergic bipolar depression. *American Journal of Psychiatry, 149*(2), 195–198.

Tohen, M., Bowden, C., Calabrese, J., Sachs, G., Jacobs, T., Baker, R., & Evans, A. (2003, May). *Olanzapine versus placebo for relapse prevention in bipolar disorder.* Paper presented at the 156th annual meeting of the American Psychiatric Association, San Francisco.

Tohen, M., Marneros, A., Bowden, C., Calabrese, J., Koukopoulis, A., Belmaker, H., et al. (2002, September). *Olanzapine vs. lithium in relapse prevention in bipolar disorder: A randomized double-blind controlled 12-month clinical trial.* Paper presented at the Third European Stanley Foundation Conference on Bipolar Disorder, Freiburg, Germany.

Tohen, M., Waternaux, C. M., & Tsuang, M. T. (1990). Outcome in mania: A 4-year prospective follow-up of 75 patients utilizing survival analysis. *Archives of General Psychiatry, 47*, 1106–1111.

Van Gent, E. M., Vida, S. L., & Zwart, F. M. (1988). Group therapy in addition to lithium therapy in patients with bipolar disorder. *Acta Psychiatrica Belgica, 88*, 405–418.

Van Gent, E. M., & Zwart, F. M. (1991). Psychoeducation of partners of bipolar-manic patients. *Journal of Affective Disorders, 21*, 15–18.

Van Gent, E. M., & Zwart, F. M. (1994). A long follow-up after group therapy in conjunction with lithium prophylaxis. *Nordic Journal of Psychiatry, 48*, 9–12.

Vaughn, C. E., & Leff, J. P. (1976). The influence of family and social factors on the course of psychiatric illness: A comparison of schizophrenia and depressed neurotic patients. *British Journal of Psychiatry, 129*, 125–137.

Volkmar, F. R., Bacon, S., Shakir, S. A., & Pfefferbaum, A. (1981). Group therapy in the management of manic-depressive illness. *American Journal of Psychotherapy, 35*, 226–334.

Wehr, T. A., & Goodwin, F. K. (1983). Biological rhythms in manic–depressive illness. In T. A. Wehr, & F. K. Goodwin (Eds.), *Circadian rhythms in psychiatry, psychobiology and psychopathology* (pp. 129–184). Pacific Grove, CA: Boxwood Press.

Wehr, T. A., Sack, D. A., & Rosenthal, N. E. (1987). Sleep reduction as a final common pathway in the genesis of mania. *American Journal of Psychiatry, 144*, 210–214.

Weissman, M. M., Markowitz, J., & Klerman, G. L. (2000). *Comprehensive guide to interpersonal psychotherapy.* New York: Basic Books.

Wever, R. A. (1984). Man in temporal isolation: Basic principles of the circadian system. In S. Folkard & T. H. Monk (Eds.), *Hours of work: Temporal factors in work-scheduling* (pp. 15–28). New York: Wiley.

Wever, R. A. (1988). Order and disorder in human circadian rhythmicity: Possible relations to mental disorders. In D. J. Kupfer, T. H. Monk, & J. D. Barchas (Eds.), *Biological rhythms and mental disorders* (pp. 253–346). New York: Guilford Press.

Wilner, P. (1995). Dopaminergic mechanisms in depression and mania. In F. E. Bloom & D. J. Kupfer (Eds.), *Psychopharmacology: The fourth generation of progress: An official publication of the American College of Neuropsychopharmacology* (pp. 921–932). New York: Raven Press.

Wirz-Justice, A., & Van den Hoofdakker, R. H. (1999). Sleep deprivation in depression: What do we know, where do we go? *Biological Psychiatry, 46*(4), 445–453.

Wulsin, L., Bachop, M., & Hoffman, D. (1988). Group therapy in manic-depressive illness. *American Journal of Psychotherapy, 42*, 263–271.

Yatham, L. N., Kusumaker, V., Parikh, S. V., Haslam, D. R. S., Matte, R., Sharma, V., & Kennedy, S. (1997). Bipolar depression: Treatment options. *Canadian Journal of Psychiatry, 42*(Suppl. 2), 87S–91S.

Yatham, L. N., Liddle, P. F., Shiah, I., Lam, R. W., Ngan, E., Scarrow, G., et al. (2002) PET study of [18F]6-fluoro-L-dopa uptake in neuroleptic- and mood-stabilizer-naive first-episode nonpsychotic mania: Effects of treatment with divalproex sodium. *American Journal of Psychiatry, 159*(5), 768–774.

Young, R. C., Biggs, J. T., Ziegler, V. E., & Meyer, D. A. (1978). A rating scale for mania: Reliability, validity, and sensitivity. *British Journal of Psychiatry, 133*, 429–435.

Zaretsky, A. E., Segal, Z. V., & Gemar, M. (1999). Cognitive therapy for bipolar depression: A pilot study. *Canadian Journal of Psychiatry, 44*, 491–494.

Index

Page numbers followed by an *f* indicate figure; *t* indicate table.

616.895
F8283

113229

LINCOLN CHRISTIAN COLLEGE AND SEMINARY

3 4711 00177 6931